MW01291256

Questions Patients Need to Ask

Meherrin Regional Library System
133 W. Hicks St.
Lawrenceville, VA 23868

Questions Patients Need to Ask

Getting the Best Healthcare

Essential Information Every Patient Needs to Know

David J. Shulkin, M.D.

A Leading Expert in Hospital Safety and Quality

610.696
S

BT
19.99
RML

39515100813803

Copyright © 2008 by David J. Shulkin, M.D.

ISBN: Softcover   978-1-4363-6759-2

All rights reserved. No part of this book may be reproduced or transmitted in any
form or by any means, electronic or mechanical, including photocopying, recording,
or by any information storage and retrieval system, without permission in writing
from the copyright owner.

Published with a Grant from the Patient Safety Officer Society, Gladwyne, PA

All proceeds from the sale of this book will benefit the Patient Safety Officer Society

This book was printed in the United States of America.

To order additional copies of this book, contact:
Xlibris Corporation
1-888-795-4274
www.Xlibris.com
Orders@Xlibris.com
48977

Contents

Dealing With Problems in the Hospital

Going Home

Dedication

To my family who continues to show me that anything is possible

And to the men and women of the Beth Israel
Medical Center who work tirelessly to serve our Patients

David J. Shulkin M.D.

List of Contributors

Michael Abiri, M.D.
Chairman Department of Radiology
Beth Israel Medical Center
St. Lukes Roosevelt Medical Center
New York, NY

Sam Acquah, M.D.
Attending Physician
Division of Pulmonary Medicine
Beth Israel Medical Center
New York, NY

David Bernard, M.D.
Senior Vice President and Chief Medical Officer
Beth Israel Medical Center
New York, NY

Brett Bernstein, M.D.
Chief, Endoscopy Services
Division of Gastroenterology
Beth Israel Medical Center
New York, NY

Catherine Binck, MSN, RN
Senior Nurse Education Manager
Beatrice Renfeld Division of Nursing Education and Research
Beth Israel Medical Center
New York, NY

Henry Bodenheimer, Jr., M.D.
Chairman, Department of Medicine
Beth Israel Medical Center
Professor of Medicine
Albert Einstein College of Medicine
New York, NY

Joann Coffin, RHIA, CPHQ
Vice President
Beth Israel Medical Center
New York, NY

Edward E. Conway Jr., M.D., M.S.
Professor and Chairman
Pediatrician-in-Chief
Milton and Bernice Stern Department of Pediatrics
Chief Division of Pediatric Critical Care
Beth Israel Medical Center
New York, NY

Gale Cantor, RN, MS, CFNP
Director of Graduate Medical Education
Beth Israel Medical Center
New York, NY

Arnold J. Friedman, M.D.
Chairman, Department of Obstetrics and Gynecology
Beth Israel Medical Center
New York, NY

John T. Fox, M.D., FACC
Director, Cardiac Catheterization Laboratory
Beth Israel Medical Center
New York, NY

Susan P. Gold, MSW
Vice President of Administration
Beth Israel Medical Center
St Lukes and Roosevelt Hospital Center
Executive Director,
Continuum Cancer Centers of New York
New York, NY

Michael L. Grossbard, MD
Associate Director, Continuum Cancer Centers of New York
Chief, Division of Hematology Oncology
Beth Israel Medical Center and St. Luke's and Roosevelt Hospitals
Professor of Clinical Medicine
Columbia University College of Physicians and Surgeons
New York, NY

Louis B. Harrison, MD
Clinical Director, Continuum Cancer Centers of New York
Chairman, Radiation Oncology
Beth Israel Medical Center and St. Luke's and Roosevelt Hospitals
Professor of Radiation Oncology
Albert Einstein College of Medicine
New York, NY

Christine Hinke, M.D.
Associate Director, Department of Rehabilitation Medicine
Beth Israel Medical Center
New York, NY

Gregg Husk, M.D.
Chairman, Emergency Medicine
Beth Israel Medical Center
New York, NY

Michael T. Inzerillo, RPh, MBA
Corporate Director of Pharmacy
Continuum Health Partners
New York, NY

Patti Juliana, MSW
Executive Director, Stuyvesant Square
Beth Israel Medical Center
New York, NY

Martin S. Karpeh Jr., M.D.
Chairman, Department of Surgery
Beth Israel Medical Center
Director of Surgical Oncology &
Associate Director Continuum Cancer Centers
New York, NY

Donald M. Kastenbaum, M.D.
Vice Chairman, Department of Orthopedics
Assistant Vice President/Medical Director Perioperative Services
Beth Israel Medical Center
New York, NY

Brian Koll, M.D., FACP
Chief, Infection Control
Beth Israel Medical Center
Associate Professor of Clinical Medicine
Albert Einstein College of Medicine
New York, NY

I. Michael Leitman, M.D.
Chief, General Surgery
Vice Chairman, Department of Surgery
Beth Israel Medical Center
Associate Professor of Clinical Surgery
Albert Einstein College of Medicine
New York, NY

Joanne V. Loewy, DA, MT-BC, LCAT
Director, The Louis Armstrong Center for Music & Medicine
Beth Israel Medical Center
New York, NY

Patricia Luhan, Ph.D.
Corporate Executive Director
Department of Pathology and Laboratory Medicine
Beth Israel Medical Center, St. Luke's and Roosevelt Hospitals
New York, NY

Bonnie Lupo, MS, SBB(ASCP)
Technical Director, Blood Bank
Department of Pathology and Laboratory Medicine
Beth Israel Medical Center
New York, NY

Kevin Maccoll, MPS, CACAC
Treatment Manager
Stuyvesant Square
Beth Israel Medical Center
New York, NY

Peter D. McCann, M.D.
Chairman, Department of Orthopedic Surgery
Beth Israel Medical Center
New York, NY

Marvin A. McMillen, M.D., FACS, MACP
Chief, Division of Surgical Critical Care
Beth Israel Medical Center
New York, NY

Woodson Merrell, M.D.
Chairman, Department of Integrative Medicine
Beth Israel Medical Center
Assistant Clinical Professor of Family and Social Medicine
Albert Einstein College of Medicine
New York, NY

Harris M. Nagler, M.D., FACS
Chair, Sol and Margaret Berger Department of Urology
Beth Israel Medical Center
Chief of Graduate Medical Education and Academic Affairs
Professor of Urology, Albert Einstein College of Medicine
New York, NY

Mark S. Persky, M.D.
Chairman, Department of Otolaryngology
Head and Neck Surgery
Beth Israel Medical Center
Professor of Clinical Otolaryngology
Head and Neck Surgery
Albert Einstein College of Medicine
New York, NY

Russell Portenoy, M.D.
Chairman, Department of Pain Medicine and Palliative Care
Beth Israel Medical Center
Professor of Neurology and Anesthesiology
Albert Einstein College of Medicine
Chief Medical Officer
Continuum Hospice Care/The Jacob Perlow Hospice
New York, NY

David Robbins, M.D.
Director, Endoscopic Ultrasound Program
Beth Israel Medical Center
Assistant Professor of Medicine
Albert Einstein College of Medicine
New York, NY

Edwin A Salsitz, MD, FASAM
Attending Physician
Chemical Dependency Unit
Beth Israel Medical Center
New York, NY

Robert Schiller, M.D.
Chairman, Department of Family Medicine
Beth Israel Medical Center
New York, NY

Michael J. Serby, M.D.
Associate Chairman
Department of Psychiatry and Behavioral Sciences
Beth Israel Medical Center
Professor of Clinical Psychiatry
Albert Einstein College of Medicine
New York, NY

David Seres, M.D.
Director, Medical Nutrition
Columbia Presbyterian University Hospital
Attending Physician
Beth Israel Medical Center
New York, NY

Vijay Shah, M.D.
Director, Blood Bank
Department of Pathology and Laboratory Medicine
Beth Israel Medical Center
New York, NY

David J. Shulkin, M.D.
President and Chief Executive Officer
Beth Israel Medical Center
Professor of Medicine
Albert Einstein College of Medicine
New York, NY

Fran Silverman, LCSW, ACSW
Director of Social Work and Home Care Services
Beth Israel Medical Center
New York, NY

Latha Sivaprasad, M.D.
Medical Director, Quality Management and Patient Safety
Beth Israel Medical Center
Assistant Professor of Medicine
Albert Einstein College of Medicine
New York, YNk

Rebecca Stalek, M.D.
Resident, Internal Medicine
Beth Israel Medical Center
New York, NY

Daniel Steinberg, M.D.
Associate Program Director Internal Medicine
Beth Israel Medical Center
Assistant Professor of Medicine
Albert Einstein College of Medicine
New York, NY

Alicia Tennenbaum, LCSW, ACSW
Department of Social Work and Home Care Services
Beth Israel Medical Center
New York, NY

Mary Walsh, MSN, RN
Vice President, Patient Care Services and Chief Nursing Officer
Beth Israel Medical Center
Corporate Chief Nursing Officer for Quality, Standards, and Practice
Continuum Health Partners
New York, NY

Kevin Weiner, M.D.
Chairman, Department of Rehabilitation Medicine
Beth Israel Medical Center
New York, NY

Bruce M. Wenig, M.D.
Chairman, Department of Pathology and Laboratory Medicine
Beth Israel Medical Center, St. Luke's and Roosevelt Hospitals
Professor of Pathology,
Albert Einstein College of Medicine
New York, NY

Deborah A. Wible, PharmD
Corporate Director of Pharmacy
Continuum Health Partners
New York, NY

James F. Winchester, M.D.
Chief, Division of Nephrology and Hypertension
Beth Israel Medical Center
Professor of Clinical Medicine
Albert Einstein College of Medicine
New York, NY

Arnold Winston, M.D.
Chairman, Department of Psychiatry
Beth Israel Medical Center
Professor of Psychiatry
Albert Einstein College of Medicine
New York, NY

Amy Wirtner, M.D.
Assistant Residency Director, Emergency Medicine
Beth Israel Medical Center
New York, NY

Stanley R. Yancovitz, MD
Chief, Chemical Dependency Division
Director of Clinical AIDS Activities
Beth Israel Medical Center
Professor of Clinical Medicine
Albert Einstein College of Medicine

Barbara Zeifer, M.D., M.B.A.
Vice Chair, Department of Radiology
Beth Israel Medical Center
Associate Professor of Radiology
Albert Einstein College of Medicine
New York, New York

Forward

My goal as chief executive of Beth Israel Medical Center is to make our hospital the safest in the world. I believe all hospital CEOs should have patient safety as their top priority.

For almost twenty years I have focused on the quality and safety of healthcare. During that time I've seen my colleagues recognize and address the gaps in best practices that perpetuate clinical errors. There have been remarkable advances in the past five years alone. Yet it is clear that we are still at the beginning of a long journey.

I've always believed that hospital safety requires an engaged and empowered patient or patient advocate. When people get sick, naturally they are scared and anxious. Because of this, patients are often afraid to speak up in the authoritarian environment of many medical centers. Sometimes patients don't even know their caregivers' names, which contributes to their reluctance to ask questions. Even physicians when they themselves are hospital patients can be passive, afraid they will be criticized for being outspoken or difficult.

Looking back upon dozens of medical errors, I see it is all too common for patients or family members to remain silent when they suspect something is wrong or improper in their care.

One example I will never forget involved a middle-aged woman who underwent an extensive battery of tests and procedures meant for another patient. After several hours of testing, an astute technician discovered the hospital had been testing the wrong patient. Fortunately, no harm was done. We learned that personnel in the admissions office had placed another patient's ID bracelet on this woman. When we asked the patient why she had responded when called by the wrong name, she replied that she thought the hospital must know what it was doing. She assumed she was being called by the name of the doctor who would be taking care of her. This seemed odd, she said, but she didn't want to offend hospital personnel.

I've seen far too many hospital patients remain in pain simply because they assumed that their doctor knew what was pain regimen was best and they were afraid to question their caregivers judgment. I've seen other patients who have received too much pain medication, and as a result had severe complications, for these same reasons. If there is one thing that I have learned in my quest to improve patient safety, it is that patients and families must be willing to leave their comfort zone and speak up.

In this book, I've tried to look at the hospital from your perspective. I've used my experience as a physician, administrator and researcher in quality and safety to ask the questions for you, the patient. I've asked the leaders in clinical thought to put themselves in your shoes and help you become an active partner in your care.

Engaged and questioning patients can be more difficult for doctors, nurses, and hospital staff to care for. But enlightened medical professionals recognize that patients need to be partners in their own care. I hope this book will encourage you to ask questions, share concerns, make suggestions and become an active member of your healthcare team. I believe it is only when you and your family are full participants that we can have the safest hospital possible.

David J. Shulkin, M.D.

About the Hospital

How Do I Use Public Information to Find the Best Care?

Latha Sivaprasad, MD

I finished my training in Internal Medicine at Washington University/Barnes-Jewish Hospital in 2002. After five years of clinical Internal Medicine in the hospital setting and multiple hospital admissions of family members in four different hospital settings, something became clear. Hospitals are prone to errors, and healthcare delivery is variable. A typical patient probably does more research on a restaurant or car than on a doctor or hospital. They might not know where to look for this kind of information. And I was probably no different.

From 2007-08, I completed a Fellowship at Beth Israel Medical Center in New York City focusing on quality improvement and patient safety. During this time, I discovered a wealth of information available to the public that I never knew existed. This is what I want to share with you.

What public data is available on hospitals and doctors?

With relatively minimal effort, it is now possible to compare the quality of care you would likely receive from a specific doctor or hospital. Organizations such as The Joint Commission (formerly the Joint Commission on Accreditation of Healthcare Organizations) and the Centers for Medicare and Medicaid Services (CMS) are taking the lead to ensure that patients are adequately equipped with the right information. The current publicly reported data allows you to analyze several items. Major examples are listed below. All website URLs and references are listed at the end of this chapter for your convenience.

Is my doctor board-certified?

You could access your state's Department of Health website (for New York *http://hospitals.nyhealth.gov/*) or HealthGrades (*www.healthgrades.com*)

How does my hospital perform in "Core Measures" or the care of problems such as pneumonia, congestive heart failure, or heart attack?

This information is available to the public. You can find this information by accessing *www.hospitalcompare.hhs.gov*

How do hospitals perform in certain types of surgeries and procedures?

Data is voluntarily submitted to The Leapfrog Group (*www.leapfroggroup.org*). You can compare how hospitals differ in their quality of delivery of medical care with procedures such as CABG (coronary artery bypass graft), PCI (percutaneous coronary intervention, AAA (abdominal aortic aneurysm), Bariatric Surgery, etc.

Do patients feel respected at a certain hospital?

There is a mandatory survey given to a sample of discharged patients after their discharge called the HCAHPS (HospitalConsumer Assessment of Healthcare Providers and Systems).

This survey focuses on the patient's experience in the hospital. Fundamental issues such as respect/courtesy, nursing, physician care, and pain control are addressed. This data is now being publicly reported on *www.hospitalcompare.hhs.gov*.

Has my doctor been sued?

This information is important to patients, and rightfully so. Some specialties such as Obstetrics have a much higher rate of malpractice than Internal Medicine so it is important to keep that in mind. The best way to allay your concerns is by discussing issues directly with your physician. You can access your state's Department of Health website (for New York *http://hospitals.nyhealth.gov/*) or HealthGrades *www.healthgrades.com*.

How do I use available information to find the best care for me?

Providing patients with the right information to make educated medical decisions is finally becoming a central focus to many national organizations and hospitals. In the past it was acceptable to just take your doctor's word for it. The culture of medical consumerism and patient-centered care is rightfully changing this approach. As a patient, you need to change with the times and take a more active part in your medical care. You need to become a self-advocate.

More than books and magazines, both the internet and word of mouth will be used as the major sources to obtain information about the quality of medical care. The "References and Resources" section at the end of this chapter will help you muddle your way through all the information that is now available at your fingertips.

What questions should I ask my doctor about the hospital?

Trusting your doctor is usually a gut feeling, but be smart and ask the right questions. Lots of information can be obtained with online searches. Some general questions to ask are as follows:

1. Who is there at night if I get sick? Is there a full time Hospitalist (Board Certified physician usually trained in Internal Medicine who is dedicated to the practice of inpatient medicine), Intensivist (Board certified physician in Critical Care), or other attending physicians in the hospital 24 hours a day?

   You want to know, especially at night, what staff is available to care for you. In teaching hospitals it is usually a combination of housestaff (doctors in training who have completed medical school and have an MD) and attending physicians (doctors who have finished their training).

2. Do you have privileges to take care of me here?

   You will want to know if your doctor will be able to provide medical care for you if you are admitted to the hospital.

3. Is this the best hospital for the condition I have?

   You will want to know if another hospital in the area has better outcomes or results for the medical condition for which you seek treatment.

4. Would you send your family to this hospital?

5. Does the hospital accept my insurance plan?

6. Is the hospital accredited by The Joint Commission?

   Usually the hospital is accredited by this national organization every three years.

7. Is this a teaching hospital?

You will want to know if there are doctors in training or doing their residency after medical school as part of your healthcare team. This usually means more up to date care but can also mean having more physicians (at various levels of training) who spend time at the patient's bedside. Patients have mixed opinions about that.

8. Does the hospital participate in public reporting forums allowing me to compare other hospitals in the area?

Public reporting by a hospital is often a way to show that the organization has commitment to the principles of quality improvement and is focused on process improvement activities.

9. What is the Nurse to Patient ratio?

This can vary greatly. In ICU settings, the ratio is usually 1 nurse for every 2 patients. On the general medical floors it can range from 1 nurse for every 3-6 patients. The lower the ratio, the more personal attention a patient is likely to receive.

10. Does the hospital have computer physician order entry (CPOE)?

Hospitals with CPOE typically have fewer errors compared to orders that are handwritten and harder to interpret.

11. What percentage of the doctors is board-certified?

Each specialty has it own dedicated "Boards," an extremely detailed exam meant to embody the standard knowledge a physician should know for practice. Older doctors may have "grandfathered" out of their Boards because they were in practice and developed clinical expertise before the exam or the specialty was created. It is important to note this difference because these physicians are exempt from this certification requirement.

How often is data updated?

Data is updated with different frequencies. For example Leapfrog data is usually submitted yearly. Core measure data outlining the standard of care with Pneumonia, Congestive Heart Failure (CHF), Acute Myocardial Infarction

(AMI), and Surgical Care is updated quarterly. It will be most useful to just access the dedicated websites as listed below and get the real-time data that is available. The databases are usually interactive for the medical consumer so that hospital comparison is user-friendly and can be easily done.

References and Resources for Patients:

- NCQA (The National Committee for Quality Assurance) *www.ncqa.org*
- The Joint Commission
  www.jointcommission.org
- Bridges to Excellence
  www.bridgestoexcellence.org
- The Leapfrog Group
  www.leapfroggroup.org
- Hospital Compare
  www.hospitalcompare.hhs.gov
- HealthGrades
  www.healthgrades.com
- IHA (Integrated Healthcare Association)
  www.iha.org
- AQA (Ambulatory Quality Alliance)
  www.ambulatoryqualityalliance.org
- AHA /HQA (American Hospital Association/Hospital Quality Alliance)
  www.aha.org/aha/issues/HQA/index.jsp
- NQF (National Quality Forum)
  www.qualityforum.org
- IHI (Institute for Healthcare Improvement)
  www.ihi.org
- AHRQ (Agency for Healthcare Research and Quality)
  www.ahrq.gov
- National Guidelines Clearinghouse
  www.guideline.gov
- CMS (Centers for Medicare and Medicaid Services)
  www.cms.hhs.gov
- OIG (Office of Inspector General)
  www.oig.hhs.gov
- NSQIP (National Surgical Quality Improvement Program)
  www.nsqip.org

Getting Admitted to the Hospital

Daniel I. Steinberg, MD

A few years ago, my grandmother fell and broke her hip. She was taken to a hospital emergency room and had to be admitted for surgery. Although her doctors and nurses were great, and she was getting excellent care, when I saw her in the ER she looked frustrated. She had a lot of questions, no answers, and this was making her upset and nervous. She didn't know how she would get from the ER to her room. She wondered who would be taking care of her in the hospital and how would she know what was happening with her care. My grandmother was taking a lot of medications at home and she didn't know if she would still be taking these while she was in the hospital. After I explained the admission process to her and answered her questions, she felt a lot more comfortable. So that you feel more comfortable during your hospitalization, here are answers to some questions you may have.

What happens when I get admitted to the hospital?
How does the admission process work?

There are a number of ways a person can be admitted to the hospital. Each is a little different, and knowing what to expect helps to make things a lot less confusing.

Direct Admission

If you are "directly admitted" to the hospital, it means that you will not go to the emergency room. Sometimes people are directly admitted from their doctor's office if it is felt that they need to be hospitalized but don't need emergency care. Patients having an elective surgery or other procedure that has been planned in advance, such as a knee replacement, can be directly admitted too. Often these patients just come to the hospital for their procedure straight from home.

If you are being directly admitted, when you arrive at the hospital, your first stop will be the Admitting Office. "Admitting", as it's called by hospital staff, looks a lot like a large doctor's office waiting room, with chairs, magazines and televisions. When you come in, you'll be greeted by the people at the registration desk. They'll take your insurance information, have you fill out some forms and give you an Admission Packet (for more on the Admission Packet, see question two, below).

I asked our hospital's admitting staff what they would want patients to know. They said, "Most of all, a patient should know that once they are here, we will take care of all the details and help guide them through the process every step of the way—they will not be left alone!"

They also wanted patients to know that there can sometimes be a short wait before your hospital bed is ready, or the operating room is ready to receive you. Although your doctor has called ahead and told the hospital you are coming and all the arrangements are being made, it still takes time to have your room cleaned and prepared for you. Sometimes the operating rooms have emergency cases, and this might be the cause of a short delay. When things are ready, you'll be escorted by someone up to your hospital room or to the operating room, where a nurse will be waiting for you.

Being Admitted From the Emergency Room

If you came first to the emergency room for an urgent problem and you need to be admitted for further care, you'll stay there, under the supervision of the ER doctors and nurses, until your hospital bed is ready. When it's time for you to "go upstairs", as we call it, a hospital transporter—someone trained in lifting and moving patients—will pick you up and bring you directly to your room, where a nurse will be waiting for you. You will be given an Admission Packet either in the ER or upon arriving at your room.

"Hand Off"—How The Transfer of Your Care Between Doctors and Nurses Occurs

In addition to just moving from one place to another, being admitted to the hospital from either your doctor's office or the emergency room involves another very important activity—the transfer of your care and information about you from one group of health care providers to another. Both doctors and nurses participate in this activity that we officially call "hand off". The Joint Commission, the agency that sets and enforces quality of care standards in the US, has asked all hospitals to implement a standard "hand off" procedure[1]. I actually wear a large button on my white doctor's coat that says "Hand Off for

Patient Safety" to help constantly remind us all how important it is to do it right for every patient, every time.

During a hand off, the doctors and nurses in the ER will talk to their colleagues on the unit you are going to, and inform them about your condition, diagnosis and any treatments that have been started. They will ask questions of each other if they have them and they'll be sure that everyone is clear on things. If you are being directly admitted from your doctor's office, your doctor will speak on the phone with the doctors who will be taking care of you in the hospital. There are often lots of details to discuss, and hand offs are always done in a very ordered and "check list" type of way, so that nothing is missed or left out.

When you are admitted, you should ask the doctors in the emergency room and then again on your unit "have you spoken with my outpatient doctor?" Timely communication between all your doctors is part of quality care, and is something you should insist on. Here's another tip I tell patients: always keep your outpatient doctor's phone number with you, even if your doctor works at the hospital you always go to. This makes it easy and fast for someone to call them if need be. Carrying your doctor's contact information with you is a simple step you can take to help make sure things get done right.

Admitting Orders

Admitting orders are a set of instructions written by a doctor that tells the nurses and other hospital staff what specific care, treatments and testing are to be done for a patient when they arrive on the unit.

A typical set of admitting orders includes the following:

- **the "service" you are being admitted to** (Medicine, Surgery, Pediatrics, Obstetrics, etc.)
- **the name of your attending physician**
- **your diagnosis**
- **your condition** (serious, stable, unstable)
- **your activity level** (whether you should stay in bed or you can walk around)
- **your diet** (low salt, diabetic diet, liquids only, nothing to eat, etc)
- **allergies to medications** that you may have,
- **how often your vitals signs are to be checked**
- **any specific blood tests that need to be drawn**
- **the medications you will be taking while you are in the hospital**
- **any special instructions for the nursing staff** (for example, how often to check your blood sugar if you are a diabetic, or what type of tests you will be going for).

It's a good idea to ask about your admitting orders and be sure you understand them.

Why should I read the information in the Admissions Packet?

The Admissions Packet contains a lot of important information. It will explain to you how the hospital works and tell you what resources and services are available.

One of the most important things in the packet is a booklet that many hospitals include called "Your Rights as a Hospital Patient". The booklet explains things like how to choose a health care proxy, how your consent for procedures is obtained and recorded, how the hospital protects your privacy, and how to file a complaint and contact the Patient Representatives' Office.

In the booklet you will also find the Patients' Bill of Rights. As a patient you have many rights and privileges that are protected by law. These Rights are yours regardless of your status as a citizen or where you live. It is very important that you read them. Being aware of your Rights as a patient is one of the first and most important ways you can participate in your own care.

Other things in the Admissions Packet include instructions on how to get telephone and television service, the hospital's visiting hours, religious services that are available, and lots of other useful information.

Who will be caring for me in the hospital?

You will be cared for by a team of healthcare professionals who will work together to give you the best and safest care possible. Teamwork is something good hospitals value, promote and practice every day. In fact it's very likely that many of the people taking care of you have known each other and worked together as a team for years. The number of people looking after you may seem confusing, but they all have important roles in your care. Some of the people you will meet are described below.

The **attending physician**, a doctor who has completed special training in their field, will be in charge of your care. The name of your attending physician is printed on your hospital bracelet and in your chart. The attending physician may also work with and supervise **residents and fellows**, who are doctors-in-training. An attending physician will examine you and discuss your care with you personally every day that you are in the hospital.

Some outpatient doctors stay in charge of the care of their patients when they are admitted to the hospital. It is also increasingly common for outpatient doctors to turn over the care of a patient to doctor who has special experience in treating hospitalized patients. These special "inpatient physicians" are called **hospitalists**. You should ask your outpatient doctor what type of arrangement they have planned for you. There's no right or wrong way, and the quality of your care will be the same with either approach. Hospitalists communicate with outpatient physicians regularly throughout a patient's hospitalization to give them updates, and work together when a patient is discharged to be sure a good follow-up plan is in place.

Physician's assistants and **nurse practitioners** are medical providers with advanced training who often work directly with an attending physician. They work in the emergency room, on the inpatient wards, in the operating rooms and in many other areas of the hospital.

Nurses on the floor will give you your medications, change your dressings, examine you, respond to your calls and requests, ask you about your pain level and do many other things for you. They work under the supervision of the **nursing supervisor**, who is the senior nurse on the floor.

Unit clerks or "ward clerks" keep track of all whereabouts of all patients on the unit, put charts together, coordinate patient movement with the Admitting Office, and are a great resource of information for patients and families about the policies and procedures of the units they work on. When you call a particular unit it the hospital, it's the unit clerk who usually picks up the phone.

Patient care assistants are people who assist the nurses and doctors in providing care. They check vital signs (blood pressure, heart rate, temperature and breathing), help patients get cleaned or changed, and assist patients in eating or going to the bathroom, and take patients for walks in the hall.

Physical therapists and occupational therapists have special training in rehabilitation. They design a personalized exercise and rehabilitation program for each patient, and then work with that patient during their hospital stay.

Social workers are experts in home care services, and how insurance plans, disability and other social services work. They help get patients to rehabilitation facilities or other long-term care facilities, and work closely with the doctors and nurses to ensure that patients are safely discharged from the hospital.

Nutritionists are available for consultation and are often called in by physicians to help decide on the right diet for a patient.

Chaplains of many different faiths are available to come to see you in your room. Ask your doctor or nurse to call them for you if you would like. In my experience, many patients find a visit from a Chaplain to be very comforting and re-assuring to them.

Patient representatives are available to you if you are unhappy with your care or anything about your hospitalization. They'll work for you, representing your interests, to try to resolve any problems or concerns you may have.

Ethics physicians are doctors who have special experience in ethical issues such as end of life care, conflicts of interest, disagreements between physicians and patients, advance directives and other areas. An "Ethics Consult" may be called by a doctor, a patient or a family member.

There are many other valued and essential members of the health care team. These include **phlebotomists** who are specially trained in drawing blood, **food service workers** who will prepare and serve you your meals, **transporters** who will take you to tests or procedures, and **environmental service workers**, who will keep your room, your bathroom and the hallways clean, comfortable and safe. Last and but most certainly not least, are our many **volunteers** who help keep the hospital running by bringing patients books, helping patients with writing letters or other tasks, and a variety of other things.

And finally, don't be surprised if while you are a patient or family member of a patient, you run into members of the hospital administration. Instead of sitting in their offices all day, our hospital leadership feels strongly that it's important to make regular "rounds" on the floors to talk to employees, patients and families to find out what the hospital is doing well, and what we could be doing better.

Will I still take the same medications in the hospital that I take at home? What can I do to be sure I get the correct medications while I am in the hospital?

Most patients who are admitted to the hospital will continue taking the same medications that they take at home. However, depending on your condition or what type of procedure you are having, some of your medications may be stopped temporarily.

The process of ensuring that a patient is given all their home medications when they are admitted—and of figuring out which medications need to be stopped—is called "medication reconciliation". It is considered one of the most important tasks that nurses and doctors must complete. The Joint Commission has made medication reconciliation a National Patient Safety Goal that all hospitals must address[2].

As a patient, you should be actively involved in the medication reconciliation process. Be sure to check and make sure that you are being given all of your outpatient medications. If you aren't receiving a medication you take at home, be sure you ask and understand why not.

You may be started on new medications, and if so you should understand what each medication is for. Two questions you should ask your doctor or nurse when you are admitted are "Have you checked to be sure that it's safe for me to take all these medications together? How do they affect one another?" and "What are the side effects of the new medications I am getting?" The more active you are in your care—especially when it comes to your medications—the less likely anything will go wrong, or you'll be unpleasantly surprised by a side effect you didn't know about.

I tell all my patients to carry an updated list of their medications with them at all times, and also to leave a copy of this list with someone they trust who can be reached in an emergency. This is one of the most useful steps you can take to ensure that you get the correct medications when you are in the hospital.

Medication reconciliation occurs again if you are transferred within the hospital, and again when you are being discharged.

Why do people keep asking me the same questions over and over? Don't people talk to each other?

When my grandmother was admitted to the hospital for a broken hip and I went to visit her, she asked me the same thing. She had just come up from the ER, was settling into her bed, and just when she was about to get some rest "another young doctor came in and asked me all the questions all over again". When I heard this was occurring, I was actually quite happy, because this told me she was in a good hospital. Let me explain.

When someone is sick, injured or under stress, it's often hard for them to remember all of their medications and their medical history. When I see patients and ask them questions they have already been asked, they will often remember very important things that they had forgotten to mention to others, such as allergies to medications or important symptoms they had been having over recent weeks.

Another reason we ask things over and over is to be sure that we haven't forgotten to ask patients about something. Although doctors and nurses are very well trained professionals, we're only human, and occasionally we might forget to ask about something. Having each member of the team caring for you ask the same questions is how we "check each others' work", so to speak. It's similar to why airline pilots—who are also very well trained, of course—each conduct the same set of checks before take off, to be sure that nothing is missed or overlooked.

In addition, during the time you stay in the hospital, the results of tests that were sent may come back, and we may need to ask you further questions, or confirm something we talked with you about previously, as part of interpreting the test results.

Do we talk to each other? Of course! This is perhaps the most important thing we do, because good communication is the essence of teamwork, and teamwork is essential for providing high quality care. Your doctors and nurses meet to discuss your care many times throughout the day. As an attending physician and a hospitalist myself, I meet with the residents and interns that I supervise every morning to discuss all the patients we are caring for together. I talk to the nurses about what their thoughts are. I speak with the social workers, the physical therapists, the nutritionists and many other people throughout the day.

In addition, throughout the week we have "multi-disciplinary rounds". This is a meeting in which doctors, nurses, social workers and physical therapists sit down together to discuss the care of all the patients on a particular unit.

What is my "white board" for?

At our hospital we use a "White Board" to help with communication between you and your healthcare team. The white board, located on the wall near your hospital bed, is a great and new tool that is starting to appear in hospitals around the country. It serves a number of important purposes.

First, it lets you know who is taking care of you. The names of all your doctors and your nurse for the day will be on there, so if you have a question, you know who to ask for.

The white board is also a way for you to express yourself to us—to let us know what's important to you. If you get cold at night and need extra blankets, write that down so we know! If you are nervous about having your blood drawn, write that down so we can talk to you and re-assure you about things. If you want a particular family member informed of things, put their name and phone number on the white board. If something is important to you, we definitely want to know about it, and putting it on the white board is a great way to tell us. If you cannot write things down yourself, someone will assist you.

Finally, the white board helps your doctors and nurses work as a team. Nurses change shifts a couple times a day, and sometimes doctors change units, too. The white board keeps us all informed of who is responsible for your care at any given time. For example, when I go into a patient's room and I need to tell that patient's nurse something, I just look on the board and I know who to speak with. Similarly, if nurses need to speak with a patient's doctor they know right away who to call. It's a great system that helps us communicate with each other and with you.

How do I stay informed about my progress and the results of my tests?

Each day, the team of doctors and nurses taking care of you will update you on things. The doctors will usually come around to see each patient early in the morning. If they have new information, they'll let you know. Sometimes your attending physician will come see you later in the afternoon and may have an update for you.

Some tests, such as an MRI or certain blood tests, can take a few hours, or even days in special cases, for the results to come back. A good habit to get into is to ask your doctor when the results will be back. This way, you aren't left wondering, and you know what to expect.

If you ever feel that you don't understand what's going on or you have a question, speak up and ask! There is always a doctor and a nurse available to come to your room and give you—or your family, if you would like us to talk with them—a progress report, or to answer questions. When my grandmother was admitted to the hospital for a broken hip, I arrived at the hospital in the middle of the night, at 3am. I was worried about her, and I had some questions. I couldn't wait until morning to get answers, as she was very sick at that point. I asked for the doctor to be paged, and she arrived at our room within a few minutes.

Here's a tip that I give to all my patients: Keep a piece of paper and a pen next to your bed and write down your questions when they occur to you. If you have your questions written down, you won't forget to ask them when the doctor or nurse comes in.

Can I read and get copies of my medical record?

Yes. If you would like to see your inpatient records while you are hospitalized, commonly referred to as your "chart", this will be arranged. Most hospitals, including ours, require that a doctor be present with you when you are viewing your chart. Having a doctor present helps you understand what you are reading and avoids any misunderstandings. In addition, most people have lots of questions when they read their chart, so this way someone is right there to answer them for you.

If you would like a copy of your entire medical record, New York State law requires that this be provided to you after you have submitted a written request to the Director of Medical Records at the hospital. The hospital may charge a small fee, but you cannot be denied a copy of your medical record if you cannot pay. More information on how to get a copy of your medical record and the fee is in your Admission Packet.

What if I want another opinion about my care?

If you would like another opinion about your care, you should express this to your attending physician. He/she can arrange for one of his/her colleagues, or a specialist in a particular area, to see you. If you are at all uncomfortable with the care you are being given, or you feel your attending physician is not respecting your wishes, you should contact the Patient Representatives' Office. Information on how to do this is in the Admissions Packet.

I've noticed over the years that hospitalized patients sometimes request a second opinion because there has been a breakdown in communication between doctor and patient, and they simply want to know what's going on with their care. Asking lots of questions to be sure you always understand your diagnosis and treatment plan will go a long way towards making you feel more satisfied with your care. If your diagnosis is unclear, as sometimes happens, your doctor should inform you of this uncertainty. Two great questions to ask your doctor that will help you understand what they are thinking are "How certain are you of my diagnosis?" and "What other diagnoses are you considering or do you think are possible in my case?" When you get the answers, write them down so you can refer to them later.

I've heard of hospitals getting two patients confused. How do hospitals prevent this? What can I do to help make sure it doesn't happen to me?

The Joint Commission has published their 2008 National Patient Safety Goals for hospitals[3], and goal number one is to improve the accuracy of patient identification. The Joint Commission's recommendation, and our practice, is to always use at least two patient identifiers when providing care, treatment or services.

At our hospital, the two patient identifiers we use are name and date of birth. In many situations you will be asked by a nurse or doctor directly to give your name and date of birth before receiving treatments or undergoing tests. If ever a patient is unable to communicate their name and date of birth, the hospital staff will check and double-check this information themselves before proceeding.

Very careful efforts are made to ensure that the correct surgical procedures are done on the right patient and at the right site (meaning, not on the wrong side or in an organ that was not supposed to be operated on). We always follow something called the Universal Protocol for Preventing Wrong Site, Wrong Procedure, Wrong Person Surgery™.

The Universal Protocol starts with what is called a "time-out". When a time-out occurs, everyone in the operating room stops what they are doing. The patient's name, the procedure to be done, the site/location and side of the body, the position of the patient, the supplies and equipment and any x-rays or tests are all reviewed and confirmed as being correct, out loud, by multiple people. The process is so strict that it must be documented on by someone as having occurred, and this documentation becomes part of the medical record.

Even with all the above safety checks in place, there are steps you can take to help ensure that you are not confused with another patient. Here are four things you can do:

1. Check your hospital ID bracelet and be sure your name and date of birth are correct.
2. Check to see that your name is spelled correctly wherever you see it in the hospital (on your chart and outside your room, for example).

3. Be sure that when you talk to your doctors in the morning, you understand the plan for the day and know what to expect.
4. Trust your instincts. If something doesn't seem right and you think you are being confused with another patient, speak up immediately. If you are about to have a test or procedure, ask your nurse or doctor to stop what they are doing, and request that a time-out be taken to check that you are not being confused with someone else.

Although the hospital is a very safe environment and the chance of getting two patients confused with each other is extremely low, being an active participant in your own care always helps to make things safer and reduce the chance of an error.

[1] http://www.jointcommission.org/PatientSafety/NationalPatientSafetyGoals/08_hap_npsgs.htm

[2] http://www.jointcommission.org/PatientSafety/NationalPatientSafetyGoals/08_hap_npsgs.htm

[3] *http://www.jointcommission.org/PatientSafety/NationalPatientSafetyGoals/08_hap_npsgs.htm*

While in the Hospital

Catherine J. Binck, RN, MSN and Mary Walsh, RN, MSN

What can I expect from my Nursing Care in the hospital?

The practice of the profession of nursing encompasses the diagnosis and treatment of human responses to actual or potential health problems through such services as casefinding, health teaching, health counseling and the provision of care supportive to, or restorative of, life and well-being. The process of nursing is fulfilled through independent function as well as through collaboration with other members of the health care team and the community.

The Department of Nursing assumes responsibility for maintaining standards for the assessment, planning, delivery, and evaluation of nursing care in a variety of settings. These standards encompass the spirit of the American Nurses' Association Standards of Practice. The Department of Nursing carries out its function in accordance with the objectives and policies established by the Board of Trustees and the Medical Center.

What do I do if I see my nurse is not washing her hands after she has been with another patient and is now coming to see me?

All of us are concerned about the risk of spreading infections from one person to another. Research has shown that the best way to reduce this risk is for everyone in the Medical Center to wash his/her hands before and after providing patient care. If at anytime you have a question about whether or not a staff member has washed his/her hands before caring for you, do not hesitate to ask the staff member to wash his/her hands. Limiting your risk of infections is more important than any embarrassment you may feel in bringing this issue up with the staff.

You will notice that the staff will use one of two methods of handwashing. If hands are visibly soiled, the staff member will wash with antibacterial soap and water. At other times, staff will use waterless, alcohol based hand gel. Dispensers containing this product are located in every patient care room, as well as by each elevator.

You can help prevent the spread of infections even more, by asking your family and visitors to wash their hands when they are visiting you.

References
MMWR: Oct, 25,2002/51(RR16);1-44
Joint Commission International Center for Patient Safety: Empowering Patient and Families about Infection Control
The Joint Commission: Speak Up; Five Things You Can Do to Prevent Infection

How can I best prevent a fall while in the hospital?

Your safety is very important to us. When you are a patient in the hospital several factors may increase your risk of falling. First, the illness that brought you into the hospital or medications you are taking may make you fell weak or dizzy, especially when you stand up. Second, medications prescribed by your physician may contribute to the problem by increasing your need to use the bathroom. Third, the hospital is a new and unfamiliar environment

When you are admitted to the hospital, your nurse will ask you a series of questions designed to determine your risk of falling while in the hospital. If you are at an increased risk, the nursing staff will check on you more frequently.

Here are tips for preventing falls while you are in the hospital:

- Familiarize yourself with your environment, including the height of your bed, the location of the light switch and the bathroom
- Ask for help before getting out of bed, or out of a chair or if you need assistance for any reason. Remember: call, don't fall!
- Get up slowly and carefully. Sit and dangle your legs over the side of the bed for a moment, especially if you have been in bed for a long time
- Ask the nursing staff to assist you in keeping everything you need where you can reach it, including your call bell, telephone and personal items
- Wear non-skid slippers or shoes when getting out of bed
- Wear your eyeglasses
- Turn the light on before getting out of bed, especially at night
- Use assistive devices such as canes or walkers when needed

Please do not:

- Attempt to get out of bed without assistance if you are not feeling well
- Lean on furniture or equipment that has wheels
- Attempt to get out of a wheelchair or off a stretcher without assistance
- Lean over the side of the bed to reach for something

Side-rails will be positioned for your support/safety based on an individual nursing assessment of your needs.

References:
Continuum Health Partners, Health Guide: Preventing Falls: Information for Patients and visitors
Centers for Disease Control and Prevention, National Center for Injury Prevention and Care: Preventing Falls Among Seniors accessed 3/25/08

Should I worry about the ratio of nurses to patients in the hospital?

Concern over your care is understandable. You should not worry about nurse staffing but if a question arises please bring the question to the attention of the Nurse Manager. Staffing guidelines are in place in this hospital and are based on Best Practice Models and the average daily patient census and the activity (nursing care needs) of every unit in the hospital. Staffing is planned in advance and validated every shift.

Are there ways that I can lessen the risk of developing a pressure ulcer?

A pressure ulcer, sometimes referred to as a "bedsore", is caused by constant pressure to the skin located over boney parts of your body such as your heels, elbows, hips, back of your head, or your sacrum (tailbone). This pressure results in the skin opening, and a wound or ulcer developing. Patients who are seriously ill, malnourished, frequently wet, and/or are unable to move around are at increased risk for developing a pressure ulcer.

When you are admitted to the hospital, your nurse will inspect your skin and ask you several questions to determine your risk of developing a pressure ulcer while you are in the hospital. Many hospitals use methods to decrease the chance that you will develop a pressure ulcer. These include: mattresses on all of our beds that reduce pressure to the skin, a daily assessment of your potential to develop a pressure ulcer, attention to your nutritional needs, and specialized treatments if a pressure ulcer does develop.

What can I do to decrease my risk?

Constant pressure to the skin only happens when an area of the body is not moved. If you are able, please be sure to change positions in bed frequently. Even a slight change in position can make a big difference. It is important to change positions frequently, even if you are most comfortable in just one position. If you have difficulty moving, the nursing staff will assist you.

When your skin is wet for long period of time, your risk for developing a pressure ulcer increases. Please let the nursing staff know immediately any time your skin is wet, either because of incontinence, perspiration or a draining wound. A nurse will work with you to develop a plan to keep your skin clean and dry.

Poor nutrition can contribute to skin breakdown. Your physician will order the diet most appropriate to your medical condition in consultation with our clinical nutritionists. Eating as much of your meals as possible and drinking plenty of liquids will help to protect your skin.

The first sign that a pressure ulcer may be developing is change in skin color. If you notice a new red or bluish/purple area, or any new wound, please alert your nurse.

References
Continuum Health Partners, Health Guide: Pressure Ulcer Prevention
Institute for Healthcare Improvement: Accessed3/25/08: Relieve the Pressure and Reduce the Harm

Is there a way to decrease my risk of getting a deep venous thrombosis (DVT) after surgery?

Deep vein thrombosis (DVT) is a condition where a blood clot develops in one of the veins deep inside your legs. It does not involve the small veins you can easily see on your legs. The blood clot that forms in DVT takes up room in the vein, and blocks the smooth flow of blood. Also, if a piece of the blood clot, referred to as an embolus, breaks off and travels through the blood stream, it can block blood flow to areas of your body such as your lungs, brain or heart, causing potentially serious damage to these organs.

One of the major risk factors for the development of DVT is a reduced blood flow through your legs caused by lack of movement. Examples of this include: being in bed during and after surgery, or sitting in a chair for long periods of time without moving your legs.

Prevention is the best medicine for DVT. During surgery we will place your lower legs in sleeves attached to a piece of equipment called a compression device. While you are having surgery, this device will alternately squeeze and release your lower legs gently, in a manner similar to what happens when you walk. This will keep the blood moving. Depending on the type of surgery you are having, your physician will order the use the compression device after surgery in the Post Anesthesia Care Area, and when you return to your room. You can make the best use of this device by keeping the sleeves on until your doctors and nurses tell you they are no longer necessary.

You can also keep the blood flowing through your legs when you are in bed, or sitting in a chair by doing some simple exercises. Tighten and release your calf muscles several times an hour or pick your feet up off the bed and make circles with your ankles.

As soon as you are able, get out of bed and walk. Nothing is better for prevention of DVT. If you are in pain, please speak to your nurse about receiving pain medication.

There are several additional factors that increase you risk for DVT. These include a family history of DVT, pregnancy, heart failure, an inherited blood-clotting disorder, some forms of cancer, obesity, taking birth control pills or hormone replacement therapy, previous surgery, or a previous episode of DVT. Please be sure to tell us if you have any of these risk factors so that we can make the best plan of care for you.

In addition, your physician may decide to order a low dose of an anticoagulant or blood-thinning medication for you. These medications work by preventing blood clots from forming.

References:
Continuum Health Partners, Health Guide: Deep Vein Thrombosis
Medline Plus Accessed 3/24/08: Deep Vein Thrombosis
Mayo clinic.com Accessed 3/14/08: Deep Vein Thrombosis

There are so many staff caring for me in the hospital. How can I keep track of who is responsible for my care?

All providers of care—doctors, nurses, technicians and even consultants—are required to wear an ID on their uniform/lab coat which is visible at eye level. Depicted is the person's name and title. In your room there is a "white board" which will let you know which resident (MD), RN and PCA is caring for you on the current shift. Your care, however, is led by an attending physician and should be noted on your ID band as a reminder. The staff can clarify this for you at any time.

Can I expect that someone is going to respond to my call bell when I need someone?

Yes, absolutely. This is one of our most important customer service goals. Your call may be answered first by a clerk (Unit Support Associate) at the nursing station but should immediately be followed up in person by one of the staff. Always tell your doctor, nurse or other staff member how you are feeling. Do not be afraid to ask for help or, for example, pain relief. Our goal is to provide excellence in patient care delivery.

What can I do if I have a concern about my nursing care?

You can ask to speak to the unit's nurse manager or on evenings/nights/ weekends you can speak to the nursing supervisor.

What if the floor is too noisy for me to get the rest I need?

Hospitals, by virtue of the care provided 24 hours a day, are busy places. However, we recognize that a healing environment is a healthy environment. Unit overhead paging is cut off at 9pm and lights are dimmed at 10pm. Please bring to the attention of your nurse any problems with noise so that appropriate steps can be taken to decrease the noise.

Resources for Nursing Care

- Unit Nurse Manager
- Web

  - American Nurses Association: *www.nursingworld.org*
  - Visiting Nurses Association: *www.vnsny.org*

- CMS (Medicare) 1-800-633-4227 or 1-800-446-2447

Medications in the Hospital

Michael T. Inzerillo, RPh, MBA and Debra A. Wible, PharmD.

Medication safety, even when medications are used in the hospital, is everyone's responsibility. Did you know that something as common as acetaminophen, the active ingredient in Tylenol (Johnson & Johnson), can be harmful, even fatal, if too much is taken? While we take medications to help us eliminate symptoms, control blood pressure, cholesterol, blood sugar, or a variety of other issues, we must take nothing for granted when using medications in the hospital setting.

To help us in that regard, we've responded to a list of questions that you, as a patient, might find important to ask during your stay at a hospital.

When I come to the hospital, should I bring a list of medications I have been taking at home?

When you come to the hospital, it would be extremely helpful if you brought a list of medications you are taking at home. This will help your doctors, nurses and pharmacists ensure three things:

1. **Continuity of care**

    In other words, you might be taking a drug at home to control your blood sugar. If that information is not communicated to your doctor upon your admission to the hospital, and if your blood sugar happens to be within a normal range when you are admitted, the fact that you require long-term control of your blood sugar might be temporarily overlooked. We say "temporarily" because blood sugar levels change rapidly and may be too high the next time it is checked.

2. **Continuity of dosing**

Very often, different people receive very different doses of the same medication. If you can only remember the name of your medication, but can't remember what dose you take or how often you take it each day, the doctor might have to prescribe a different dose when you are first admitted to the hospital. This might be more important in some situations than in others, especially if you are taking medication for a thyroid condition, heart disease, blood pressure control or bipolar disorder.

3. **Allergy Check**

Sometimes the medication you take at home might provide a clue to your doctor that you are allergic to a certain medication or group of medications. Avoiding drugs to which you may be allergic is extremely important as we will discuss later.

At a minimum, when you are admitted to the hospital, you, a family member or caregiver should be able to tell your doctor the name and strength of your medication and the number of times you take it each day.

Should I tell my doctor about over-the-counter or herbal medications I might be taking?

Yes. First, this will help the doctor better understand your full range of medical issues. It will give your doctor the opportunity to ask why you are taking these medications or supplements, and it may provide an opportunity to prescribe a more appropriate medication. Also, herbal medications may not be as harmless as people may believe. Some herbal medications have significant drug interactions and may need to be discontinued while you are in the hospital.

While you are in the hospital you should only take the medication prescribed by your doctor and administered by your nurse. The nurse maintains a complete record of the medication you have taken and the time you have taken it. Taking over-the-counter medications or herbal supplements on your own while you are in the hospital may change your clinical condition, such as your blood pressure or laboratory values. This may lead to further, and sometimes unnecessary, testing. Remember, everyone is working as your team while you are in the hospital, and you are the center of that team.

How do I know I am not getting someone else's medications?

While you are in the hospital, you can be confident you are receiving medication prescribed for you and only you. First, your doctor, physician's assistant or nurse practitioner will prescribe a medication specifically for you. They select the drug, dose, route of administration (i.e., by mouth, by injection, etc.), the number of times a day you should receive the drug, and the times of the day that you should receive it. This is all based on your clinical condition alone. They work to ensure that every medication you receive is absolutely necessary—nothing is given "just in case."

Next, a pharmacist receives the order from the prescriber and checks it to ensure it is accurate and complete. Your prescription, or medication order (as it is called when you are in the hospital), is then entered into your specific medication profile. The medication profile is a list of all medications each patient is receiving when in the hospital. It helps us make sure people are receiving only those medications intended for them.

The medication profile also serves as the nurse's medication administration record. This is the list the nurse uses to make sure the right patient is receiving the right drug.

How can I prevent getting the wrong drug or wrong dose in the hospital?

A common rule within the nursing community but remembered by all practitioners is the Five Rights, which states:

> **"The right medication, at the right dose and the right route,
> for the right patient at the right time."**

In addition to the steps taken as we discussed earlier, this rule helps everyone ensure that there is no confusion in medication use. However, this important rule can be made stronger if everyone, including the patient, starts remembering and working with a Sixth Right:

> **"For the Right Reason"**

When a nurse brings a medication to you, please ask, "What is this medication and why am I taking it?" Several medications have more than one reason, or indication, for use. Sometimes, the dose of that one medication may differ significantly when used for different reasons. The following table highlights some important drugs with different reasons for use at different dosage levels:

Drug Name	Indications	Doses
Lovenox (enoxaparin—Sanofi-Aventis)	• Prevent blood clots before abdominal surgery • Prevent blood clots before knee replacement surgery • Prevent blood clots before hip replacement surgery • Treat blood clots in the hospital • Treatment following a heart attack	• 40 mg injection once daily • 30 mg injection every 12 hours • 30 mg injection every 12 hours or 40 mg injection once daily • 1 mg/kg injection every 12 hours or 1.5 mg/kg injection once daily (with warfarin) • 1 mg/kg injection every 12 hours (with aspirin)
Methotrexate	• Severe psoriasis • Severe, active rheumatoid arthritis • Various types of cancer	• 10 to 25 mg weekly • 7.5 mg once weekly • 15 to 30 mg every day
Heparin	• Treatment following a heart attack • Irregular heartbeat—Prevent blood clots • Blood clot prevention	• Up to 5,000 units to start, then up to 1,000 units/hour • 5,000 units to start, then 20,000 to 40,000 units per day • 5,000 units injection every 8 hours
Megestrol Acetate	• Breast cancer • Muscle-wasting associated with AIDS	• 40 mg orally four times a day • 800 mg daily
Methadone	• Pain management • Addiction treatment	• 2.5 mg to 10 mg every 8 to 12 hours • 80 to 120 mg once daily
Azithromycin	• Treatment of community acquired pneumonia • Prevention of endocarditis	• 500 mg daily for 7 days • 500 mg once

| Trimethoprim-Sulfamethoxazole | • Urinary tract infection treatment | • 2 tablets every 12 hours for 10 to 14 days |
| | • Urinary tract infection prevention | • 1 tablet twice weekly |

Most hospitals in the United States use a Drug Formulary, which is a list of all drugs approved for use within the hospital. Because there are tens of thousands of drug products available for use, a hospital cannot possibly stock every drug. The Drug Formulary lets all health care providers know which drugs are routinely stocked and available for use within the hospital, and which products might have to be changed to an equal but different product.

This might impact you during your hospital stay if you receive a brand name drug at home, but a generic equivalent product is stocked and used in the hospital. For example, you might take Zocor (simvastatin—Merck) 10 mg once daily at home; this is a peach-colored tablet. If the hospital uses generic simvastatin, the nurse might give you a white tablet instead. The two tablets will look different, but you can be confident the dose and the drug (or active ingredient) is the same. Remember, this is an excellent time to ask the nurse what this medication is and why it looks different than what you take at home. The only bad communication is no communication—talk to your nurse, doctor or pharmacist regularly during your hospital stay.

The Joint Commission is an organization that sets standards of care for hospitals in the United States. The Joint Commission also helps us meet those standards by issuing guidelines and alerts. One of those guidelines addresses the use of Look-Alike/Sound-Alike Drugs.

As you may already know, many medications have names that look or sound alike. To address this issue and ensure we don't confuse any medication with one another, hospitals use TALLman LETTERing when prescribing, profiling, dispensing and administering these drugs that look and sound alike. This type of lettering helps everyone make sure we are always selecting the right medication. The following are some examples:

Tallman Lettering	Brand Name	Generic Name	Reason for Use
celeBREX	Celebrex	Celecoxib	Pain
celeXA	Celexa	Citalopram	Depression
metRONIDAZOLE	Flagyl	Metronidazole	Infections
metFORMIN	Glucophage	Metformin	Diabetes
zyPREXA	Zyprexa	Olanzapine	Schizophrenia
zyRTEC	Zyrtec	Cetirizine	Allergies

Another issue the Joint Commission helps us with is High Risk/High Alert Medications. This is a list of medications that may have a higher level of risk associated with their use and, therefore, require a greater level of attention. The following are examples of High Risk/High Alert Medications and the steps taken to ensure their safe use:

High Risk/High Alert Medication	Steps Taken to Ensure Safety
Concentrated Electrolytes	• All concentrated electrolytes are removed from floor stock • Premixed, standard solutions for potassium chloride are purchased • Highly concentrated sodium chloride is stocked in the pharmacy only
Enoxaparin	• All orders require indications for use
Insulin	• Doses must be prescribed in UNITS: "U" is a prohibited abbreviation • Insulin products are dispensed on a patient-specific basis only • Insulin products are dispensed in color-coded safety devices

Finally, the Joint Commission has helped hospitals develop programs where at least two different types of patient identification are used every time you are approached to either take a medication, have blood drawn or undergo any type of procedure. In addition to reading your identification bracelet, which every patient receives when they are admitted to the hospital, your nurse might also ask you your name or use some other form of identification just to "double check" the right patient receives the right treatment.

How do I know I won't receive a drug to which I am allergic?

You, the patient, play a very important role in making sure you do not receive a drug to which you may be allergic. First, as we discussed earlier, the list of medications you take at home, before you are admitted to the hospital, is very important, not only in alerting the doctor as to what medications you are taking, but also in providing an idea about what you should NOT be taking. You may be taking one type of antibiotic instead of another because you may be allergic to penicillin. The fact that you are taking erythromycin or tetracycline may give the doctor reason to ask why you are taking that instead of penicillin.

Then, the doctor would have the opportunity to ask you what exactly happens when you take the medication to which you are allergic. Sometimes expected side effects, such as upset stomach, are mistakenly referred to as an allergic reaction. Every opportunity to have open communication about your past medication use makes it easier for your health care team to make sure you receive the best therapy from this point forward.

Next, once a medication order (prescription) is written, that order is placed on your medication profile. In addition to relying on the pharmacist's professional expertise in identifying real or potential allergic reactions, every hospital should have an electronic system that checks every medication order for both drug allergies and drug interactions. Your pharmacist will alert your doctor and nurse of the need to change any medication order that may present a problem.

Although you might not have one yourself, you may notice other patients wearing a red wrist band in addition to their identification bracelet. The red wrist band is a visual alert that the patient is allergic to one or more medications; food and other allergies (i.e., latex) may be listed there as well. Your nurse will check the red wrist band every time she is about to give you a drug to make sure you are not allergic to it.

If you do have a red wrist band, which signals an allergy, you can help everyone by reminding the nurse about your allergy every time she brings you a medication.

How do I know I am going to get the right prescriptions when I go home?

Believe it or not, the job of making sure you are going to get the right prescriptions when you go home starts when you first come into the hospital. The technical term for letting your doctor know all about the medications you are taking at home is "Medication Reconciliation." The list of medications you provide is checked against the doctor's reasons for prescribing different medications for you. If the doctor, nurse or pharmacist determines you are receiving a drug you have no reason to take, that medication will not be continued. Also, it might be determined that you have a reason for taking new medication and that new medication will be started when you are in the hospital. Finally, the dose of your medication may change while you are in the hospital.

For these and other reasons, the medications you are to take when you go home may be very different from the ones you took when you came into the hospital. Your doctor will prepare prescriptions for you to take with you when you are discharged from the hospital. You should review these prescriptions very carefully with your doctor, nurse or pharmacist. You are encouraged to ask any questions about new medications and about whether or not you should continue taking your previous medications.

When do I need to ask to speak to a Pharmacist in the hospital?

You can speak with a pharmacist anytime during your hospital stay. Some hospitals have a Drug Information Center staffed by a pharmacist. Ask your nurse if your hospital has a Drug Information Center and ask for the telephone number.

Other hospitals may have pharmacists working on or near the patient care units. Just ask your nurse or doctor how you can contact your hospital pharmacist. Finally, some hospitals actually have a retail or community pharmacy located within the hospital where you may elect to fill your discharge prescriptions. Just like the pharmacist at your local drug store, your hospital pharmacist is a valuable resource.

What are the medication resources I can consult?

There are a variety of resources available to you regarding your medications. Here is a brief list of textbook and internet-based resources:

1) Physicians Desk Reference 2008 (PDR) (*www.PDR.net*) (published by Thompson Healthcare)
2) Consumer Drug Reference 2008 (published by Consumer Reports in conjunction with the American Society of Health-System Pharmacists)
3) Complete Guide to Prescription & Nonprescription Drugs 2008 by H. Winter Griffith and Stephen Moore
4) *www.drugs.com*
5) *www.rxlist.com www.nlm.nih.gov*
6) *www.fda.gov*

Preventing Infections

Brian Koll, M.D.

Many of us know of a family member or close friend who has developed an infection while in the hospital. Our first thought is, "How could this happen?" We forget that many patients in the hospital are admitted with infections, have weak immune systems or need invasive devices such as needles and catheters, and that not all infections are preventable.

Hospital associated infections affect an estimated 2 million patients each year.[1] Fortunately, 30% are preventable.[2] Many hospitals in the United States are working hard to keep you safe by reducing infection rates through adoption of practices endorsed by the Centers for Disease Control and Prevention, Institute for Healthcare Improvement, New York State and New York City Departments of Health, as well as participating in regional initiatives sponsored by the Greater New York Hospital Association and United Hospital Fund.

Most hospitals like ours have a Department of Infection Prevention with specially trained staff who are certified in infection prevention. Their job is to work with and for you to keep you safe, thus reducing your risk of getting an infection while in the hospital. Our ultimate goal is to have zero hospital-associated infections.

How can I help prevent infection in the hospital?

Observe the hospital staff that treat you. The single most important way to reduce hospital infections, according to the Centers for Disease Control and Prevention, is for your doctor, nurse and anyone else that cares for you in the hospital to wash their hands with soap and water or use alcohol-based hand rubs before and after treating you.[3] This is called hand hygiene. Look to see if hospital staff are practicing this hand hygiene before and after treating you.

Gloves are not a substitute for hand hygiene. Hospital staff who wear gloves without first practicing hand hygiene will have contaminated the gloves that come into contact with you. In addition to practicing hand hygiene, healthcare providers should always put on a fresh pair of gloves before caring for you and remove them afterwards. They should not leave your room wearing gloves!

Should I ask caregivers to wash their hands?

Many of us at our hospital wear a button on our lab coats or uniforms that says, "Ask me if I've washed my hands". Don't be afraid to speak up and ask your caregiver to wash his or her hands. Before they treat you, ask them if they have cleaned their hands with soap or water or used the alcohol based hand rubs. This applies to everyone: doctors, nurses, transporters, social workers, etc. None of us will be upset by this question and want to assure you that we believe in and practice good hand hygiene!

Should I worry about getting infections from other patients in the hospital?

No. In addition to practicing good hand hygiene, caregivers keep shared equipment clean and disinfected. Between patients, they wipe their stethoscopes with alcohol, clean blood pressure cuffs and other shared equipment such as stretchers and wheel chairs with a disinfectant. As with hand hygiene, don't be shy to ask if the stethoscope or equipment has been wiped down with a disinfectant before it is used on you.

What is a "bundle?"

While in the hospital you may have a catheter, a surgical procedure or need a ventilator to help you breathe. All procedures have a risk of infection and all procedures have protocols in place to reduce your risk of a catheter infection, surgical site infection or ventilator associated pneumonia. These protocols are known as bundles—these practices are bundled together because they've been proven to reduce infections.[4] By bundling instead of practicing each component separately, we can ensure maximum protection for you. There are practice bundles to prevent bloodstream infections from intravenous catheters, surgical site infections and ventilator-associated pneumonias. Compliance with the bundles is monitored and 100% adherence is expected.

What should I know about catheter care?

Many patients require an intravenous catheter (IV) and some require special IV catheters called central venous catheters also known as CVC or PICC lines. These lines are placed in an aseptic or sterile manner. Your skin will first be disinfected with betadine or chlorhexidine. The nurse or doctor will wear sterile gloves. For central venous catheters a sterile gown, mask and hair covering are also worn.

If you have an IV, the site should be clean, dry and covered with a transparent dressing. The IV will be changed every four days to reduce your chance of getting an infection known as phlebitis. If the IV site dressing becomes loose or wet, tell your nurse and he or she will replace it. Also tell your nurse if your IV line starts leaking or if you develop pain or swelling in your arm.

If you have a central venous catheter, antibacterial impregnated or coated catheters and a special antimicrobial patch placed on your skin at the catheter site are used to reduce your risk of blood stream infection. As with an IV, the site should be clean, dry and covered with a transparent dressing. The dressing is changed every few days. If the site dressing becomes loose or wet, tell your nurse and he or she will replace it. At our hospital, we follow a group of evidence-based practices known as the "Central Line Associated Bloodstream Infection Prevention Bundle" which has been endorsed by the Centers for Disease Control and Prevention and Institute for Healthcare Improvement to prevent blood stream infections from these catheters.[5]

How can I prevent an infection if I have a urinary catheter?

40% of hospital-acquired infections are urinary tract infections.[6] If you have a urinary catheter to drain urine, our hospital places the catheters in a sterile manner and uses silver-coated infection prevention catheters to reduce your risk of a urinary tract infection. If you start feeling urinary discomfort, ask your doctor or nurse to check if the catheter is clogged.

The risk of a urinary tract infection increases if the catheter is left in place for longer than three days. If your catheter is in place longer than three days, ask your doctor if you still need it. There may be other options such as an adult diaper or bedpan. Although they may sound unappealing, they may be safer than continued exposure to a urinary catheter.

If I am on a ventilator what can be done to prevent pneumonia?

Hand hygiene, the proper use of gloves, sterile supplies and equipment remain the cornerstone of infection prevention. Additionally, our hospital follows a group of evidence-based practices known as the "Ventilator Associated Pneumonia Prevention Bundle" which has been endorsed by the Institute for Healthcare Improvement to prevent ventilator-associated pneumonias. The bundle consists of doing the following:

1. Keeping the head of your bed elevated 30 degrees or higher
2. Providing daily assessments and reductions in sedation to determine if you are ready to breathe on your own and no longer need a ventilator
3. Giving medications to prevent peptic ulcer disease and clots in your legs while on the ventilator[7]

When should I have prophylactic antibiotics ordered in the hospital?

Antibiotics can be used to both treat and prevent infections. When used to prevent infection they are known as prophylactic antibiotics. Prophylactic antibiotics are most often ordered as part of the "Surgical Site Infection Prevention Bundle." You will receive prophylactic antibiotics within one hour before your surgery and the antibiotics will be stopped within 24 hours in most cases. Given properly, antibiotics can greatly lower your chances of getting a surgical site infection.[8]

Why do doctors put me in an isolation room and why do care givers wear gloves and gowns when caring for me?

Precautions are followed by staff when caring for all patients in the hospital to prevent the spread of infection from one patient to another. These are known as universal precautions and means that we practice hand hygiene for all patients and wear gloves when drawing blood and a gown if you need help with going to the bathroom. This protects you from infection and prevents the staff from exposure to blood or body fluids.

Some illnesses such as chickenpox, tuberculosis, influenza, drug-resistant bacteria which you may know as "super bugs" such as MRSA or methicillin resistant Staph require additional precautions.[3] If needed, an isolation/precautions sign will be placed outside your room or at your bedside. The sign does not list your illness but tells staff and visitors about precautions to prevent the spread of disease.

Are there statistics about my risk of infection in the hospital?

There are statistics about your hospital's and doctor's infection rates. You have every right to ask and should not be afraid to ask. You can obtain information on the quality of hospital care at the Hospital Compare website at *http://www.hospitalcompare.hhs.gov*. New York State will begin public reporting of surgical site infection rates and central line associated bloodstream infection rates in 2008.

What can I do to reduce my risk of infection while in the hospital?

Remember, you are part of the infection prevention team. There are many things that you can do to reduce your risk of getting a hospital-associated infection:

- Wash your hands frequently or use alcohol-based hand rubs, especially after using the bathroom and before eating
- Get a flu shot every year and ask your doctor if you need the pneumococcal vaccination to prevent a certain type of pneumonia
- Don't take antibiotics unless you really need them. Misuse of antibiotics can cause you to be infected with "super bugs" that are resistant to therapy
- If you are a smoker, consider a smoking cessation program. This will reduce the chance of developing a lung infection in the hospital
- If you have diabetes, discuss with your doctor how best to control your blood sugar as high blood sugar increases your risk of developing an infection.

What are the references I can use to reduce my risk of infection?

www.jointcommission.org/PatientSafety/SpeakUp
www.hospitalinfection.org
www.StopHospitalInfections.org
www.cdc.gov
www.ihi.org

References

1. Centers for Disease Control and Prevention (CDC). Monitoring Hospital-acquired Infections to Promote Patient Safety—United States, 1990-1999. MMWR, 2000; 49: 149-153.
2. Burke JP. Infection control—A Problem for Patient Safety. N Engl J Med, 2003; 348: 651-656.
3. Centers for Disease Control and Prevention (CDC). Guideline for Isolation Precautions: Preventing Transmission of Infectious Agents in Healthcare Settings 2007.
4. Berwick DM. The 100,000 Lives Campaign: Setting a Goal and a Deadline for Improving Health Care Quality. JAMA, 2006; 295: 324-327.

5. Centers for Disease Control and Prevention (CDC). Guideline for the Prevention of Intravascular Catheter Related Infections. MMWR, 2005; 51 (No. RR-10).
6. Association for Professionals in Infection Control and Epidemiology, Inc. APIC Text of Infection Control and Epidemiology: Urinary Tract Infections. APIC, 2005; 2nd Edition: 25-1-25-15.
7. Centers for Disease Control and Prevention (CDC). Guidelines for preventing health care-associated pneumonia. MMWR, 2003; 53(No. RR-3).
8. National Surgical Infection Prevention Project. Antimicrobial Prophylaxis for Surgery: An Advisory Statement from the National Surgical Infection Prevention Project. CIC, 2004; 38: 1706-1

Requesting a Consultation

David Robbins, M.D., Rebecca Stalek, M.D.,
Henry Bodenheimer, Jr., M.D.

Should I request a specialist care for me or is it better for my family doctor or internist to admit me to the hospital?

The best answer to this question depends on the reason you are entering the hospital. The advantage of having a "primary care provider" goes far beyond having a physician coordinate your ongoing and preventive health care as an outpatient. This primary physician knows your history (or your health issues), what medications you take, and most importantly best understands your overall condition when compared to your usual state of health. Your primary physician assesses the severity of your illness and decides if hospitalization is needed. This knowledge allows medical care to be tailored to what will be most effective in dealing with your particular situation.

Your physician also knows your usual physical ability, what social support you have in place, and how effective or tolerable any previous treatments may have been in the past. This information is crucial in assessing your severity of illness as you enter the hospital and helps expedite your care and get you on the road to recovery.

The example of tolerability of prior medications is particularly helpful. For example, most medical records report to what medicines you are "allergic", but many times medications that were poorly tolerated or ineffective are not described. Your primary physician is the quarterback of your healthcare team, and this role applies to your care both outside of and inside the hospital.

The role of the primary physician is not however unlimited. Medicine is a vast discipline and no one individual can be an expert on the innumerable disorders that may afflict you. Your physician may call in specialized consultants to assist in finding out what is wrong or in fixing the problems you are having.

These specialists are expert in specific disorders or treatments, but they are not necessarily experts on you. This is where the primary physician can again help to apply specialty advice to your particular situation.

It is not unusual to see more than one consultant in some cases, and good medical judgment is needed to plan what is best for you. Or you may have several conditions which, while not seemingly related to the reason you were admitted, could affect the way you are treated. You may, for example, have been advised to have a procedure to remove a small colon polyp (colonoscopy), but subsequently you develop a blood clot in your leg that requires you to start a blood thinner. The medication for the blood clot, warfarin, may make the chance of bleeding greater when having the colon polyp removed. Your primary physician can interact with the specialists to determine the risks involved, the duration of recommended treatments, and the urgency of intervention. In this example, the small polyp may be removed after the blood thinner is discontinued. If, however, the polyp shows signs of being more dangerous, the use of warfarin may be interrupted, and the polyp removal accomplished with the use of other more easily reversed blood thinners without delay.

Although it is very comforting to have the support of your "quarterback" primary physician, there are times when your problem is best handled with the expertise of a specialist. In this situation, the problem may be most quickly identified and fixed if the expert specialist is in charge of your care. Your primary physician can supply background information and expect to be kept informed of the results and treatment plan, particularly when you leave the hospital. An example of when a specialist may best be in charge is when you are admitted for a complex procedure requiring hospitalization. Here the care is directed at a particular problem. An alternative situation where a specialist may appropriately oversee your hospital admission is when you have a pre-existing problem that has been followed and managed by the specialist. An example may be if you are otherwise well but have long-standing inflammation of your bowels (colitis). This condition has required you to be under the care of a specialist gastroenterologist for years. If you developed a sudden worsening of this condition, you may be admitted to the hospital by the specialist who would be best prepared to perform tests and order treatments that would address your immediate problem.

Given all the various types of physicians that could be involved in your care, the best way to decide what is best for you is to ask direct questions. Your primary physician should recognize when your problem is largely limited to one specialty area and best handled by a specialist. Conversely, the specialist should also recognize when your total medical care is sufficiently complicated to best be directed by the long-standing primary physician. An open discussion allows clear lines of communication to be established and helps to assure that you will be getting the best care.

When should I have a specialist see me?

The field of medicine is extremely complex, and the continuous improvements in technology and experience available to deal with medical problems makes it impossible for any one individual to be expert in all aspects of healthcare. Primary physicians are experts on you and are able to provide preventive care, treat common medical problems, and assess your severity of illness when presenting with new symptoms. The primary doctor recognizes the type of problem and then decides if in-depth help would be helpful. The decision to call in a consultant is recognition that a specialist will bring added value. This value may be in the evaluation of your condition or in the precision of defining your problem. Many illnesses have various treatments, which may vary depending on the severity or classification of the illness. The addition of a specialist to your medical care team is not to make up for a deficiency of your primary provider but rather recognition by your primary doctor that special information exists and may impact the outcome of your healthcare.

A specialist should be called in whenever more information is needed. This is most important in illness that is serious and could result in disability or prolongation of your hospital stay. For less serious questions or those not impacting your hospitalization, specialty consults are best obtained as an outpatient after you leave the hospital. An orthopedic surgeon may see you for long-standing back pain or a gastroenterologist perform a routine screening colonoscopy after discharge.

Direct discussion with your primary admitting doctor will help determine if a specialist consultation is desirable. Ask for updated information on the nature of your illness, its expected course, and what treatment options are available. You should learn if different treatments are available, if they have differing side effects and which are expected to work better. Ask if you have any personal factors that would modify the course of disease or help choose among treatment options.

As you work through this information with your primary doctor, the need for more information may be identified. You can then explore with your admitting physician what type of specialist can best supply the information or technical expertise needed to get you better.

The choice of specialist is also complex, and even within a specialty some doctors have narrow areas of expertise. Among gastroenterologists (stomach and intestine experts), for example, some are expert at complex technical procedures while others may be best at treating inflammation of the intestines. Your admitting doctor may also give insight into who would communicate best with you and who might accept your insurance plan.

Since the purpose of calling in a specialist is to enhance the capabilities of your medical care team, communication among your providers is very important.

The specialist should be aware of the specific questions that led to him or her being called in and address these concerns.

The addition of a specialist often adds complexity (and cost) to your medical care, but this is to your advantage when the expertise or information provided allows better control of your illness. Expert treatment, particularly when provided early, may improve the long-term consequences of your illness and provide a valuable resource to your medical team.

Is it okay to ask my doctor for a second opinion?

The most important outcome of your care while in the hospital is that you receive the best care possible. The professionalism of your doctors demands that this is the goal and is to be achieved by using all available resources. Medical decision-making is complex, and at times, the many options available can be confusing and even frustrating. The involvement of multiple physicians, including primary care providers, specialists, house staff and even doctors covering for you after hours will no doubt generate many opinions for your care. A "second opinion" is different than a routine specialist consultation. The specialist is often called in to supply information or expertise not available through your primary care team. The "second opinion" is called in to either confirm a suggested diagnosis or course of action or to propose an alternative approach.

Second opinions are in fact routine when confirmation of serious complex decisions are desired. An example may be the resection of a tumor of the liver. Many aspects of decision making in this case may be reviewed and confirmed or modified. Does the tumor, for example, need to be removed? Should this be done surgically or can a less invasive method be used? If a surgical approach is to be used, how large a piece of liver needs to be removed? Where is the best place to do this surgery? Who is the best doctor for my problem?

A routine second opinion in such a case allows refinement of the therapeutic plan. Your primary care provider can help you assess the options of the first and second consultants and help formulate the best treatment choices. There are cases where you desire a second opinion because aspects of care are missing from your proposed plan. Or the original consulting specialist has not been able to satisfy you or your primary physician with regard to critical aspects of your diagnosis or treatment plan. This may be because the specialist is not the proper choice and does not have the expertise needed to best address your particular medical problem. Or the consultant may not have communicated well or has not gained your confidence.

Remember you are the focus of this medical consult, and you deserve to understand your situation and the options available to you. Although medicine is complicated, most issues can be explained in a direct straightforward manner using plain terms so that you and your family understand what is being discussed. If you do not feel satisfied, you should discuss this with your primary physician—the second opinion is an option open to you if concerns remain. Some patients are hesitant to ask for a second opinion because they fear "hurting the feelings" of their primary consultant. Remember medical care is designed to satisfy your health care needs, not those of your doctor. Open communication between patients across the entire health care team helps achieve the best possible care for you.

Frequently Utilized
Services in the Hospital

Care in the Emergency Department

Gregg Husk, M.D. and Amy Wirtner, M.D.

"Always wear clean underwear, because you never know when you may end up in the ER."

Are there better ways to prepare for your visit to the Emergency Department (ED)? Popular TV shows portraying EDs are entertaining but often unrealistic. Because EDs sometimes appear chaotic, what is routine to us may be confusing to you or your family. Understanding how we provide emergency care may help you prepare for your ED visit. There are 300 million people living in the US, and Americans made 100 million ED visits in 2006. It's really just a matter of time before you find yourself in our space, either as a patient or as a patient's visitor.

How do Emergency Departments (EDs) work?

Most patients who come to the ED want to "see the doc, get treated and go home." The days of house calls by Marcus Welby are over. Modern EDs rely upon nurses, radiology staff, ED techs, nurse practitioners, physician assistants and doctors to ensure our patients get state of the art care. Emergency care has become increasingly dependent upon laboratory and imaging technologies. In our nation's EDs, more than half of our patients receive a blood test or imaging procedure (most often an x-ray). These advances in care sometimes allow us to resolve problems that used to require a brief hospitalization, but increased complexity also means that an ED visit may take longer.

Our Emergency Departments are part of the nation's health safety net, and we continue to care for new patients even when we have 2 or 3 times more patients than treatment spaces. How do we ensure that the sickest patients get timely care, at times when we cannot evaluate each patient immediately? A registered nurse evaluates each patient soon after arrival, so that patients who need immediate medical attention are promptly identified. This process, called "triage," is used by EDs even when they are not overwhelmed. In EDs that have a variety of treatment locations, the triage nurse will send the patient to the most-appropriate treatment area. Upon occasion, the triage nurse may initiate certain tests (x-rays or lab tests) to expedite ED care.

After triage, you will be brought to an area to be treated. If there are no available treatment spaces and if the triage nurse has not identified a need for immediate treatment, you may be asked to wait in the waiting area. Once in a treatment room, patients are seen by both a primary nurse and a provider. The provider may be a physician in training (a resident), physician assistant, nurse practitioner, or a physician. The nurse and provider will ask you questions, perform a physical assessment, order tests they deem necessary, and provide you with information and advice. If a resident sees you, you will also be seen by an attending physician. The average patient spends less than 5 minutes in triage and less than 30 minutes with the ED provider, so knowing the types of questions we will ask will help you receive superior emergency care:

- *Know your medications* or carry a piece of paper in your wallet or purse that lists your current medications. A patient's medications are incredibly important in helping us to provide you with excellent care, and there's nothing more frustrating to us than hearing "I'm taking a little blue pill" for my heart. If you carry a medication list, make sure that you modify it each time your medications change.
- If you do not consistently take all of your medications, let us know! If you do not take 100% of your pills, you are not alone. Most people miss some of their pills, and some people fail to take many doses. Knowing about the medications that you are actually taking helps us a lot.
- Know your primary care provider and let us know their name and contact information. If we are able to reach your doctor, we'll do a better job in diagnosing your condition, and your provider will know the results of our evaluation.
- Know your health problems so we can do a better job of diagnosing and treating you. Some patients carry a list of their medical problems on the same paper that lists their medications, which is very helpful to us.

Here are the most common questions that patients ask about ED care:

If I have time before coming to the ED, what do I need to do to bring?

If possible, bring the medical information detailed above. If you have an insurance card, bring that, too, as it will help route the bill to your insurance carrier. You do not need to bring clothing or personal possessions, even if you think you may be admitted. When patients bring valuables, possessions or medications, we generally encourage their family to take these things home.

Why does an ED visit take so long?

ED overcrowding sometimes makes it difficult for us to attend to each patient in a timely manner, even though that is our goal. EDs tend to be busier in the afternoon and evening, so seeking care earlier in the day (if you have a choice) may reduce your visit length. The ED staff may be reluctant to estimate your wait—most often, because we do not know the answer. Sometimes a test takes longer than average or a particular test result may require additional testing. If you are admitted, it's possible that you may have to await a hospitalized patient's discharge, prior to a bed being available for you.

Who is in charge of my care when I am in the ED?

Your ED provider is in charge of your care. Some tests can be ordered by your triage or primary nurse, but your ED provider is responsible for your care. EDs have led the nation in having senior (attending) physicians in the ED at all times. Many patients are treated by a nurse practitioner or a physician assistant, and in teaching hospitals, patients may initially be seen by a resident. If you are not certain who is directing your care, ask to speak with your provider or the ED attending physician.

Can I have visitors with me?

Most EDs welcome visitors—having a friend or family member usually improves our understanding of your illness, and helps to ensure that our advice is well-understood. Nonetheless, when EDs are overcrowded, we may ask family members to stay in the waiting room, so we may provide space, care and privacy for all patients. Although some EDs have more restricted visitation policies, most EDs value a family member's presence. Most Emergency Departments allow parents to be present during their child's care.

What happens if I am being sent home when I don't feel ready?

Emergency care is not perfect, and it's possible that your ED provider does not fully understand your concerns, the nature of your illness, or the impact of your illness on your ability to function at home. Explain your concerns to your ED provider, and ask why they are confident that home treatment is right for you.

Also ask for the signs that should prompt you to return for further evaluation. If you still believe that you should not be discharged, ask the ED provider to speak with your primary care provider.

How do I get copies of my lab test results or my x-rays?

The medical records department not only helps us get prior information on our patients—it also helps patients to get copies of their records or test results. If you want to make sure your primary care provider knows the results of your ED evaluation, ask your ED provider to call your provider.

Fellows, Residents, Interns, Medical Students: A Teaching Hospital

Harris M. Nagler, M.D., FACS and Gale Cantor, RN, MSN, CFNP

What is a "Teaching Hospital?"

The term "teaching hospital" is generally applied to institutions that train physicians in various specialties of medicine. The best teaching hospitals have many training programs in different specialties. The ACGME (Accreditation Council for Graduate Medical Education) is the organization that monitors training programs and grants accreditation or approves teaching hospitals and specific programs. Of course, institutional leadership and educators provide constant supervision of all doctors in training.

Who is going to take care of me?

Every patient in a teaching hospital has an attending physician who is responsible for their care. An attending physician is a doctor who is licensed to practice medicine independently and has completed both medical school and post graduate medical training. Postgraduate training is the period after medical school when doctors learn how to take care of patients under the supervision of an attending physician. This period of training lasts from 2 to 8 years. The length of this training depends on the specialty.

What are these doctors in training called?

It depends. They have been called "interns." An intern has graduated from medical school and is in their first year of post-graduate training. But now the word intern has fallen out of favor. Currently, most hospitals use the term "resident." Often the term resident is used to describe someone who has completed one year of training (internship). However, most doctors training in a hospital are now called residents. A person is considered a resident until they have completed the required training for a specific specialty; different specialties require different number of years of training before a resident graduates and is eligible for certification as a specialist.

I have heard some doctors called "fellows." What does this mean?

A "fellow" is a person who has completed residency training and is continuing their training in a subspecialty field within an area of specialization such as medicine or surgery. Cardiology and endocrinology, for instance, are subspecialties of internal medicine and breast surgery is a subspecialty of surgery.

Is a resident a medical student or a doctor?

Residents are not medical students. They have completed college and medical school and are doctors who are in medical training programs.

Why would I want doctors who are in training involved in my care?

Doctors in training (residents and fellows) bring many advantages to patients and their families. Doctors in training are required to continually read and learn about the latest in medical knowledge and techniques, bringing you the most up-to-date care. Doctors in training are members of the team taking care of you, monitoring your progress and being there for you and your loved ones.

Are teaching hospitals better than non-teaching hospitals?

Yes! Teaching hospitals attract the best and the brightest attending physicians because they want to work with young talented physicians and improve medical knowledge and care. Well-known teaching hospitals also attract the best physicians in training. Large teaching hospitals, such as New York's Beth Israel Medical Center, also care for large numbers of patients. Research shows that the care is better and patients are better off in hospitals which care for many patients with similar problems. One of the best parts about being in a teaching hospital is having doctors around to care for you at all times.

How do I know who is really responsible for my care in the hospital?

Every patient in a teaching hospital has an attending physician who is responsible for their care. All interns, residents and fellows are supervised by your attending physician. Make sure that you know the name of your attending physician. At many hospitals there are signs by each bed indicating the names of your attending physicians and nurses. This makes it easier for you and is evidence that the hospital is interested in assuring that each patient knows who is ultimately in charge of their care.

How do I know that these "doctors in training" know what they are doing and are not just practicing on me?

Doctors in training have already had a lot of education and practice in medical school. They continue to learn every day by reading, going to lectures, practicing on simulators (models), and more. Importantly, every activity they perform is supervised by more experienced physicians and attendings. The attendings are responsible for your care.

What should I do if I want someone more experienced to discuss my care with?

Just ask! You can always speak with the attending physician who is responsible for your care. Remember you can always look at the boards by your bedside to remind you of his/her name. Don't be shy—it is your health and you need to have all your questions answered and your concerns listened to by your doctor.

Aren't residents overworked and too tired to care for me properly?

Many states now have laws in place to make sure this does not happen. The organization that approves training programs also has rules that prevent doctors in training from being overworked. The laws state the number of hours a doctor in training may work a day without getting a break, the maximum number of hours a trainee may work a week and require that every trainee gets at least one day off a week. Each department, as well as the institution's administration, has policies describing what a trainee should do if they are too tired and need to rest. There is always a back-up physician available to relieve the tired resident. We take resident work hours very seriously and regularly monitor work hours to be certain that residents are adequately rested.

How do I know if a resident physician has enough experience to perform a procedure on me?

Residents must prove to their supervising physicians that they are able to perform a procedure well before they can be performed by the resident.

Being in an Intensive Care Unit

Marvin McMillen, M.D., FACS, MACP

Which patients belong in an intensive care unit?

Intensive care units provide a very high level of nursing care as well as a coordinated team of physicians, pharmacists, respiratory therapists and nutritionists for patients with immediate life-threatening illness. Therefore, patients in shock from bleeding or an overwhelming infection, patients with coma, lung, heart, liver, or kidney failure will have a much better chance of surviving their illness if they are admitted to an intensive care unit.

How are the services provided in intensive care units different from routine nursing units in a hospital?

Intensive care units provide beat-to-beat monitoring of heart rate, rhythm and any evidence of coronary ischemia. They also provide breath-to-breath assessment of the adequacy of the oxygenation of the lungs and the delivery of oxygenated blood to the tissues. Blood pressure and urine output are monitored every 15 to 60 minutes. Most intensive care units have on-site ability to measure blood acid, carbon dioxide, oxygen, potassium, calcium and hemoglobin within two minutes.

For post-operative patients with heart or lung disease, intensive care units have the ability to quickly address major fluid shifts, bleeding, or deal with pain-control issues which may impair breathing or levels of consciousness. Intensive care units can also care for complex drains, unusual wounds and aspects of the surgical procedure unfamiliar to floor nurses.

For unstable patients with bleeding, intensive care units have the ability to rapidly replace fluids, red blood cells and clotting factors (resuscitation).

For patients experiencing a heart attack or heart failure, they provide drugs to improve heart function, stabilize heart rate and rhythm and maintain blood pressure. For patients unable to breathe on their own, they provide artificial breathing (ventilators.) For patients with life-threatening electrolyte or kidney abnormalities, they provide rapid artificial kidney services (dialysis). For patients in coma, they keep the heart, lungs and rest of the body working while the cause of the brain dysfunction is identified and treated.

As the American population becomes older and patients more likely to have several illnesses simultaneously, intensive care units also provide a process of care which allows safe and rapid treatments of several concurrent problems, such as hemodynamic insufficiency requiring heart and blood pressure support, respiratory insufficiency requiring a ventilator, and kidney failure requiring dialysis.

Are critical care and intensive care synonymous?

Yes.

What do ICU, MICU, SICU, CT-ICU, NICU, PICU, and CCU stand for?

Doctors and Nurses often use abbreviations that you may not be familiar with. ICU stands for Intensive Care Unit, MICU stands for the Medical Intensive Care Unit, SICU stands for the Surgical Intensive Care Unit, CTICU stands for the Cardiothoracic Intensive Care Unit, NICU stands for the Neonatal Intensive Care Unit, PICU stands for the Pediatric Care Unit, and CCU stands for the Cardiac Care Unit.

How are these units different from Cardiac Care Units?

Cardiac care units (CCUs) mostly care for only coronary artery disease (heart attack), heart failure and heart rhythm disorders (pacemakers.) CCUs work very closely with cardiac catheterization laboratories and cardiac surgeons. Intensive care units are generally more multidisciplinary than CCUs, which mostly take care of heart-related issues.

What is a special care unit?

Many community hospitals, which do not have enough patient volume to support staff for the individual units described above, have a shared unit which functions as a CCU, a medical ICU and a surgical ICU.

If I am admitted to a hospital with pneumonia, an ulcer, or for colon cancer surgery, and am transferred to an intensive care unit, who's in charge of my care?

In most hospitals today, a medical, surgical or anesthesia intensivist is in charge of your care. These individuals are trained in their basic medical discipline of internal medicine, general, trauma or acute care surgery, or anesthesia, and then obtain a further one to four years of training in critical care.

What is "board certification?"

At the conclusion of their three to five years of residency in medicine, surgery or anesthesia, doctors take an exam prepared by a national organization of experts in their field. For doctors who then do a fellowship in a further area of specialization, there may be a second exam for that further specialization. Therefore, most intensivists are board-certified in their primary specialty (internal medicine, general surgery or anesthesia) with a second exam and certification in critical care. In addition, doctors must take at least 50 hours per year of continuing medical education in their primary and specialty field, and take another exam every ten years to maintain their board certification.

Most hospitals require board certification of their intensivists.

What's an "attending physician?"

When a doctor joins the staff of a hospital, he or she submits their training, recommendations and work history in what is known as a "credentialing" process. They are then approved to take care of certain illnesses and perform certain procedures, but must continue to report their results and participate in the hospital "quality improvement" process.

From a legal point of view, an attending is the person in charge, as designated by the hospital, and the individual responsible for overseeing residents, physician assistants, nurse practitioners, nurses, respiratory therapists, nutritionists and other staff.

From an intensive care unit point of view, the primary care doctor, cardiologist, oncologist, gastroenterologist or surgeon who admitted the patient to the hospital is the "admitting attending." The intensive care unit doctor in charge is also an attending, as may be the consultants who evaluate an ICU patient for a problem in their areas of expertise. Residents and fellows are not attendings, and do not make any major decisions on ICU patients without first discussing them with the attendings.

Who are the members of the critical care team?

In addition to the intensivist in charge of the unit, most intensive care unit nurses are "Critical Care Certified" as CCRN. This means that they are familiar with the illnesses and conditions necessitating critical care, the technology of the unit itself, and the complex issues, such as end-of-life decision-making, which happen more frequently in an ICU than on routine floors.

If the hospital is a teaching hospital, there will also be residents and fellows from one to six years out of medical school. If the hospital does not train residents and fellows, there will be nurse practitioners and physician assistants.

In addition, there will be respiratory therapists, pharmacists, nutritionists and technicians who manage artificial kidneys.

What is the role of my primary care physician or surgeon in my intensive care unit care?

It varies. Many primary care physicians today assign the routine care of their hospital inpatients to "hospitalists"—internal medicine doctors who are full-time at the hospital. In the care of such patients, the ICU team is pretty much in charge of the care, and coordinates the consultation and recommendations of heart, kidney, liver, gut, endocrine, and infectious disease specialists.

In surgery, it's a bit different, as there are things the surgeon knows from the operating room that are still relevant to the ICU care. The model of care in surgical ICUs is more "concurrent"—with the ICU team providing 24 hour bedside care and support for all organ systems, but with the surgeon still involved in the issues which involve the surgery itself.

How are the decisions made in an intensive care unit?

Every day, usually in the morning, the ICU team reviews the brain, lung, heart, liver, gut, kidney, endocrine and nutrition status of the patient. The salt and water balance, infectious issues and drug interactions are all discussed. A conclusion is reached about where the patient is globally, what further tests or consultations would be useful and a plan of care established for the next 24 hours. As both illness and recovery can evolve quickly in intensive care unit patients, most ICU teams also make evening rounds.

Isn't having a breathing tube (being intubated) and being on a breathing machine (ventilator) painful?

Surprisingly not (the author has been intubated and on artificial ventilation while fully awake four times). But when the tube comes out, the patient may have a sore throat for several days. When you take a normal breath, the diaphragm descends, the pressure in the lungs decrease and the air is drawn in through the mouth or nose. A breathing machine is the exact opposite—air is blown into the lungs. If the settings on the breathing machine are incorrect or the patient not properly sedated, such intubated patients may have a tendency to struggle and be uncomfortable as they first get used to the machine. Usually a bit of relaxant (sedative) and pain reliever (analgesia) will assist comfort as the correct settings are achieved.

How can I communicate if I have a breathing tube and I cannot speak?

At the time of admission to intensive care units, many patients are waking up from surgery or have just experienced an event such as placement of a breathing tube that necessitates heavy sedation. But research has shown that prolonged sedation and intubation are not good for intensive care unit patients. Modern ICUs usually try to "wean" the patient off the ventilator and back to breathing on their own as soon as possible. So generally, as soon as you're awake with your pain properly controlled, and your lungs and strength okay, the breathing tube and the ventilator will be removed.

For the fairly small number of patients who require prolonged intubation, the ICU team uses clipboards and written notes.

Very few patients remember the ICU phase of their illness, even those who seem to be awake and interactive for days. Critical illness is associated with production of a number of "neurotransmitters" (brain messenger substances) which cause a twilight state and are usually associated with amnesia for the acute phase of their illness.

What is "life support?"

Critical Care has sometimes been dubbed, "the provision of care, the immediate removal of which would place the patient at an immediate risk of dying." In a sense, all medical care is supporting life, but if the ventilator (breathing machine) or the medications which support blood pressure or the dialysis which is correcting shock or electrolyte abnormalities were removed, death would be certain.

The issue of continuing the care often comes up, such as: "My father wouldn't want to be kept alive on life support." A better and more accurate way of communicating among families in discussions about this issue would be "Would you want full care in an intensive care unit if there was only a slight chance of recovery?"

What is the "stress response?"

When the human body is injured, there is an intrinsic system to respond to the stress of injury. This involves substances described as "adrenaline" and "cortisol." There is also a major shift in metabolism to make and preserve glucose (sugar) and redirect protein production to those proteins most important to healing. Even the most carefully done surgery elicits a stress response, though it varies with the magnitude of the surgery and the site.

There are some surprises in this stress response—a three-hour colon operation is more stressful than an eight-hour brain operation. Abdominal surgery, for some reason, appears to be particularly stressful.

While the stress response is helpful in terms of permitting the body to withstand injury, it may also be harmful. Increased blood clotting ability may inadvertently trigger blood clots in the legs or pelvis, which may break off and travel to the heart and lungs. Increased coagulation plus adrenalin produced as a part of the stress response may cause coronary artery narrowings to occlude, resulting in a heart attack. Most ICU patients will be on blood thinners and drugs that slow and protect the heart to counteract these effects.

The stress response also results in rapid muscle breakdown, which is probably responsible for much of the tiredness and weakness many people complain of when they leave the ICU. Early use of nutrition, either by nasogastric ("N-G") tube or intravenously can help ameliorate this muscle breakdown.

What is shock?

All cells in the body need oxygen for normal function, and that oxygen gets there when hemoglobin in the red blood cells picks it up in the lungs, and the heart pumps it out to the tissues. Shock is defined as inadequate oxygen delivery to support cellular metabolism to the peripheral organs (brain, heart, muscles, kidney, liver and extremities). Usually, the blood pressure falls in this state, but some patients with low blood pressure may not be in shock. So blood pressure alone is an inadequate criterion to determine shock, though pale or blue skin color, low urine output, high heart rate, and biochemical tests of venous oxygen and blood acid may be helpful.

A number of things cause shock, including blood loss in injury or internal bleeding, fluid loss in severe diarrhea, burns or heat stroke, impaired heart function from either cardiac muscle or valve dysfunction, loss of blood vessel tone due to toxins from infection and inflammatory substances produced as the body resists the germs causing the infection, release of allergic substances, external toxins or gases, and neurologic injury.

Treatment of shock varies with the underlying cause. In hypovolemic shock of blood or fluid loss, the treatment is blood or fluids (called resuscitation). Cardiogenic shock may require trying to open or bypass the coronary artery whose insufficient blood flow is resulting in heart dysfunction. If a valve has suddenly become regurgitant resulting in cardiogenic shock, open heart surgery may be necessary. Rarely, fluid can collect around the heart and cause cardiogenic shock. However, this fluid can be removed with either a needle or with surgery.

If blood pressure has fallen because of a drug or toxin, that substance must be removed, or support must be provided while the patient "metabolizes" the substance or drug. If blood pressure falls because of an allergic response, steroid drugs can be used to decrease release of the allergic substances which other drugs increase the blood pressure and a ventilator improves oxygenation in the lungs. If a spinal cord injury or other brain problem has caused neurogenic shock, drugs can be provided which mimic the normal nerve signal to maintain blood pressure.

What is "sepsis?"

The outside of the human body and the inside of most of the gastrointestinal tract is colonized with nearly 10,000 different types of germs. But only a few of these cause human illness, or are considered pathogenic organisms. Physicians divide the organisms into gram positive organisms which take up a special stain and are usually round, and gram negative organisms, which do not take up the stain and are usually shaped like short rods or boxes. But despite the prevalence of these organisms, the skin and the gut lining protect us from having the organisms enter our body and causing infection.

When germs do enter the skin, or areas of the gastrointestinal tract prone to infection (the gallbladder, bile duct, appendix, and diverticuli of the colon), some weakness of the barrier function or protective mechanisms has occurred. Sometimes we form stones in the gallbladder or appendix. Once infected, it is very hard to sterilize with antibiotics alone. So recurrent infection occurs.

Normally, the human body is very good in walling off infection with a combination of immune, inflammatory and protein substances which confine the infection to one area. An abscess will often form in the absence of antibiotics, though antibiotics can cure some abscesses without surgical incision or drainage.

But if an infection begins to overwhelm the body's defenses, the patient may become unstable with increasing heart rate, lowered blood pressure and need for more intravenous fluid. The substances being formed in sepsis may cause the small blood vessels in the tissues (the capillaries) to leak, and edema (swelling) begins to occur. This hemodynamically unstable state is called sepsis, and results from a combination of exotoxins produced by gram positive organisms and inflammatory products produced in response to gram negative organisms. Untreated with fluids, antibiotics and drainage, sepsis can lead to multiple organ failure syndrome.

What is "multiple organ systems failure (MOSF)" or "multiple organ failure (MOF) syndrome"?

As infection overwhelms the body's protective defenses, the affects on the patient can range from confused to comatose, with deteriorating kidney, pulmonary, cardiac, liver and coagulation function. Sepsis with multiple organ failure has a much higher death rate than infection and sepsis that are caught early before other organ failure develops. This is why speed is so important in the initiation of treatment in infection and sepsis. While outcomes vary based on age and other illnesses, half- to three-quarters of septic patients with multiple organ failure will die.

What is respiratory failure?

Blood picks up oxygen in the lungs to then carry it to the tissues. Respiratory failure means that the diaphragm, chest wall, air sacs in the lung (alveoli), or blood flow within the lungs are not working properly. Lungs often accumulate fluid in shock or sepsis, and intensivists often speak of the lungs being "wet." (The same thing can happen with heart failure, but that is related to increased pressure in the lung blood vessels).

Respiratory failure leading to a need for intensive care may be from muscle weakness from pain-killing drugs or diseases that weaken the muscles. It can also occur secondary to pneumonia (from germs within the air sacs), atalectasis/collapse (from the air sacs collapsing from infection or injury), pulmonary emboli (when blood clots from the legs or pelvis break off, and pass through the right heart and out into the lung arteries), and acute lung injury, which can be from aspiration of stomach acid, overwhelming infection and massive requirement for blood and blood products.

In respiratory failure, it is necessary for a machine to breathe for the patient. This ventilator has essentially three elements: a tidal volume, which is the amount of air breathed per breath; a respiratory rate, the number of breaths per minute; and the fraction of inspired gas that is oxygen   normally 21% in the air all around us, and up to 100% for a sick patient on a ventilator.

The ventilator substitutes for the patient's diaphragm and chest muscles, but it cannot substitute for the air sacs in the lung itself. That is why treatment of respiratory failure has two objectives: to support the lung function to the limits of the machine, and to identify and treat the underlying etiology of the lung failure.

What is medical futility?

The diagnosis of medical futility is both simple and complex. The simple definition is that when medical care has no reasonable chance of returning a patient to a level of functionality that they would consider acceptable, care is considered medially futile. Medical futility is a medical diagnosis, not a legal one.

From a practical point of view, we define futility as, when no member of the senior staff has ever seen a patient in a similar position recover, or when a computer search of the entire English language medical literature (a program called PubMed) has never reported a survivor in such a situation. But state laws guiding what to do once medical futility is diagnosed vary widely, with some states permitting termination of care at that point and other states only allowing the physician to so advise the family.

A classic example of medical futility is the patient with lung cancer who becomes comatose from lung cancer metastases to the brain. This individual has no chance of returning to life of any quality before the acute event occurred. And to the extent that he or she is aware of any pain, all critical care is really doing is prolonging their dying, without hope of benefit for the pain they do experience. But some states permit physicians in such circumstance to withdraw care as medically futile, while others permit families to continue insisting that this scarce and expensive resource be utilized even though it will not change the outcome.

Can my family stay with me at all times that I am in the ICU?

Many hospitals have 24-hour access for family members of critically ill patients. But more importantly, ICU's answer the phone 24 hours a day. In many ways, having a close loved one in an ICU is harder than being the patient in the bed—the combination of uncertainty, confusion and exhaustion are overwhelming. We advise families to visit often but if possible to limit the number of family at the bedside to 1-2 people in order to not overwhelm their family member.

The difficult decisions that close family members and health care proxies are often asked to make on behalf of the patients are never easy, and exhaustion from poor sleep in the waiting room chair only worsen the process. It is far better to be at the bedside as much as personally comfortable, get as normal as possible a pattern of rest at home, and call back to the unit to check up anytime of the day or night.

How can I tell if the ICU is providing high-quality care?

The intensive care unit's attending physicians should be board-certified in critical care or cardiology. A majority of nurses should be CCRNs (which means they have achieved further certification in critical care). There should be full-time intensivists in the hospitals daytimes and 24-hour coverage by board certified attending physicians to answer all emergency calls.

The professional organization of intensivsts is called the Society of Critical Care Medicine. Most medical societies are divided into groups according to specialty and profession, so doctors are in one society and nurses are in another. The Society of Critical Care Medicine has taken a different approach, and welcomes all individuals involved in critical care. Thus doctors, nurses, pharmacists, nurse practitioners, physician assistants and respiratory therapists may all participate in this group. Furthermore, this society has created a two-day course—the Fundamentals of Critical Care Support (FCCS)—for all individuals who work in ICUs.

A group of large employers who were concerned about finding a high level of care for their employees has formed an association called The Leapfrog Group. The Leapfrog Group requires that all its member institutions have their ICUs run by intensivists, with computerized doctor's orders to avoid mistakes and 24 hours a day, seven days a week coverage by intensivists and FCCS certified caregivers, who have been certified in Fundamental Critical Care Support by the Society of Critical Care Medicine. Their website is: *leapfroggroup.org*

What are the resources for patients and family in the ICU?

Critical illness is about the family as well as the patient being sick, and usually significant resources are available to help patients and families. Critical illness is depressing, exhausting and isolating. There is a natural tendency to think that no one has ever gone through this before, and chances of returning to one's pre-illness life are very poor. In fact, the opposite is true—most patients today have a 90-98% chance of leaving the intensive care unit to return to their state of health before the critical event occurred.

Most well-functioning intensive care units encourage questions and understand the need to catharse. The ICU teams also recognize scenarios such as "the out-of-town prodigal son who arrives after dad's been in the ICU for two weeks and reacts to his own grief and guilt by blaming everyone around him." The intensivist or the unit director is usually available for daily bedside updates or, if necessary, family meetings to define issues and plans.

ICU teams work closely with social workers, rehab staff, psychologists, and "healing environment staff" to try and create continuity of care for both the patient and family, whether it is in the expectation of full recovery or as part of the ritual of saying goodbye.

Laboratory and Pathology Services in the Hospital

Bruce M. Wenig, M.D., Patricia Luhan, Ph.D.,
Bonnie Lupo, MS, SBB(ASCP), and Vijay Shah, M.D.

What can I do if I feel that the person drawing my blood has missed my vein too many times?

In general, the laboratory does not oversee the draw of blood for in-patients. In clinics and outpatient centers there are patient service centers run under the supervision of the Laboratory. Phlebotomists are the technical people in the patient service centers trained to draw blood. As a general policy but not any standard policy, phlebotomists should attempt to draw bloods twice. If they cannot get the specimen after two times, someone else (generally someone with more experience) should try once. If the second person cannot get the blood, a physician should attempt to draw the blood which may require the more difficult procedure of drawing blood from an artery (arterial stick). If a phlebotomist too often fails to draw bloods, they are required to be retrained.

If I need a blood transfusion how can I assure that I get the right blood for me?

In order to assure that a patient receives the "right blood for me" the Blood Bank in the Department of Pathology maintains strict adherence to all regulatory guidelines set forth by the American Academy of Blood Banks (AABB), the New York State Department of Health (NYSDOH) and the Federal Drug Agency (FDA). Oversight begins from the moment of blood collection to the administration (transfusion) of blood.

The Standard Operating Procedures for the Blood Bank include strict policies for specimen collection, and the typing and cross-matching of blood. There are numerous checks and balances in place to assure that the "right" blood products are prepared and that the patient receives the "right' blood for him/her. A thorough review by the Blood Bank Staff is required for all transfusion orders and product pick-up to assure that the correct product(s) are prepared and dispensed. Further, face-to-face review at the Blood Bank dispense window occurs by the Blood Bank Staff with the "pick-up" staff to review all pertinent information, including patient identification information, patient's blood type and blood product's blood type occurs. At the bedside prior to any transfusions, two staff members are required to "sign-off" verifying patient identification information, including the patient's complete name, medical record number compared with the wristband, as well as verifying the product(s) requested, and verifying blood type of the blood product to that of the recipient before administering any blood product(s).

Checks and balances include the reporting of all errors. Any error must be reported to the Blood Bank, prompting an immediate investigation and, if needed, notification of the involved parties. All internal blood bank errors are reported to the FDA as required by the Blood Product Deviation reporting regulations. Additionally, there is on-going internal Quality Assurance (QA) monitoring in the blood bank.

What is the role of the pathologist and the laboratory in patient care?

"I thought pathologists only did autopsies and worked with dead people?" This is a common refrain heard by pathologists from laypeople. While other physicians may understand the role pathologists play in the overall management of patients, the layperson may view pathologists as laboratory assistants to the physicians who "really" make the diagnosis.

The pathologist and the laboratory play a vital role in the care and welfare of the patient. The pathologist is the primary diagnostician for all tissues sampled and/or removed, including cytology preparations (e.g., PAP smears), fine needle aspirations, biopsies and removal of larger specimens (e.g., colon, stomach, lung, liver, uterus, prostate, etc). Pathologists who specialize in the evaluation of tissue specimens are anatomic pathologists and more specifically are collectively referred to as surgical pathologists. Although functioning "behind the scenes" removed from direct patient care, the pathologist is an integral member of the clinical team that is administering to patients with cancer/tumors, as well as patients with non-cancerous conditions. The pathologist's role is multifactorial. In the simplest of terms, it is the pathologist's job to look into a microscope and to make the correct diagnosis of the sampled tissue(s). However, that "final" goal is not an isolated achievement nor is the diagnosis the sole responsibility placed on the pathologist. There are numerous factors that go into the diagnosis of cancers and non-cancerous lesions/conditions. Relative to cancer diagnosis, it is the pathologist who determines the type of cancer (e.g., carcinoma, lymphoma, melanoma, sarcoma, etc), how invasive is the cancer, has the cancer spread (metastasized) to lymph nodes or other body sites, has the cancer been completely removed, and are there any pathologic findings that may allow for predicting the behavior of the cancer. As needed, there are additional studies/tests that are performed under the responsibility of the pathologist to assist him/her in the evaluation of diseases. Some of these tests include special staining (e.g., immunohistochemistry) and molecular diagnostics (e.g., fluorescent in situ hybridization [FISH] for Her-2).

The clinical pathology laboratory oversees the testing of body fluids (e.g., blood, serum, urine), including chemical analysis (e.g., sodium, potassium, glucose, etc) and hematologic analysis (e.g., red blood cell count, white blood cell count, hemoglobin, clotting times, etc). Other aspects of clinical pathology laboratory include testing for infections (microbiology) and the blood bank (see above). With some exceptions, the majority of the testing in the clinical laboratory is performed on automated analyzers. These analyzers process the test fluid(s) and through complicated processes produce an array of numbers for each specific test ordered. Specialists in clinical pathology maintain oversight of the clinical laboratory testing, in general, with specific responsibilities assigned for each discipline of the clinical laboratory (i.e., chemistry, hematology, microbiology, blood bank).

When are second opinions from a pathologist a good idea when looking at tissue specimens?

Second opinions in pathology may be initiated by the patient or by the patient's clinician. In addition, if you have had a diagnosis made at one hospital and you are being referred to or you seek a specialist at another medical center, it is a requirement of the second medical center to review (i.e., give a second opinion) the outside surgical pathology slides before definitive treatment of the referred patient(s). Second opinions in pathology are primarily intended to affirm a diagnosis, especially although not limited to complicated diagnostic cases, and to minimize clinically significant errors that have a direct impact on patient care. Although the overall percentage of affected cases is not large, the consistent rate of discrepant diagnosis uncovered by second opinion surgical pathology may have an enormous human and financial impact. This quality assurance practice has been threatened in the era of managed care and cost containment.

Can I get copies of my pathology reports?

Yes, copies of your pathology report are available through your clinician or through the Department of Pathology. Appropriate verification is required in order for the Department of Pathology to release your report. The pathology report is the document that contains the pathologist's diagnosis for a surgical or cytologic specimen. The pathology report not only contains your diagnosis but also may include important information about the prognosis of your disease. The pathology report is a legal document that becomes a part of your medical record.

When should I ask to speak to a pathologist?

Nearly all medical decisions are based upon the results of the laboratory. These results can be complicated and written in highly technical language. The patient that is able to understand their laboratory result is in a better position to make an informed decision regarding their medical care. The pathologist is the physician producing these results; these results are conveyed to your clinician who shares that information with you. The pathologist very rarely communicates with the patient. You might consider speaking to a pathologist to discuss your diagnosis or a family member's diagnosis. The critical role that the pathologist plays in your diagnosis coupled to the limited resources for the patient to interpret their own pathology report represent potential reasons why you might consider contacting (by telephone, email or in person) a pathologist.

Resources for Patients

American Academy of Blood Banks Website—AABB.org.
College of American Pathologists Website—cap.org.
Kronz JD, Westra WH, Epstein JI. Mandatory second opinion surgical pathology at a large referral hospital. Cancer 1999;86:2426-35.
Manion E, Cohen MB, Weydert J. Mandatory second opinion in surgical pathology referral material: clinical consequences of major disagreements. American Journal of Surgical Pathology 2008;32:732-7.
Shitibata PK Website—www.thedoctorsdoctor.com.

Radiology Services in the Hospital

Michael Abiri, M.D. and Barbara Zeifer, M.D., MBA

The chances are very high that at some point during your hospital stay you will have an encounter with the Department of Radiology. The interaction may take place at your bedside with portable equipment, or you may be transported to the radiology department. The test may take a few minutes or possibly hours. You will meet the radiology technologist who is responsible for producing your images, and possibly a radiology nurse. On occasion, you will meet and speak with the Radiologist. A Radiologist is a highly specialized medical doctor who supervises and directs all aspects of your examination. The radiologist establishes protocols, assesses and interprets the images and then generates a report. The radiology report details all the findings that the Radiolgist has made during a careful review of the pictures, and directs your doctor to the significant abnormalities, he or she then concludes by providing a specific diagnosis whenever possible. Very often there are 2 or more diagnoses that can look the same; in that case, the Radiologist will offer what is called a "Differential Diagnosis" meaning the list of possible diagnoses that fit the findings seen on your radiographic images. If an additional exam can help pinpoint your diagnosis more accurately, that test will be recommended. Once it is generated, this report can be viewed by all physicians participating in your care.

The Radiology Department may seem as a large, confusing and hectic place, with many events going on at once. This can be understandably intimidating, unnerving, and at times frightening. Understanding two key facts will help you feel more comfortable during your stay in Radiology:

1) Every single radiology staff member (even those not directly involved in your care) wants you to have a positive experience in his or her department. That means you can approach any of them with questions or concerns of any sort; and

2) The Radiologist (whether you meet them or not) is YOUR doctor also, responsible for your care and safety throughout your stay in the department of Radiology.

The following are the most common questions and concerns that patients will have when they visit any radiology department:

How can I be sure I am having the exam that my doctor ordered for me?

There are many different types of Radiology exams that can be ordered, including: plain X-Rays, Computed Tomography (CT), Magnetic Resonance Imaging (MRI), Ultrasound, Nuclear Medicine, and vascular-interventional procedures (VIR) which include image guided biopsies and catheter angiograms among other things.

Your doctor will directly order the specific Radiology exam he or she wants you to have either into the hospital's information system or on a special request form on paper, and often will call to discuss this with the Radiologist as well. Your name then immediately appears on the appointment list for that area of Radiology, for that day. The Radiology department will then coordinate with your nursing staff an appropriate time to perform your test. The radiology technologist will print up an information sheet pertaining to your exam and will make sure it is clear. About an hour before radiology is ready to perform your exam, the technologist will arrange for you to be brought to Radiology and soon after that a transporter will arrive and you will be on your way.

When you arrive in the appropriate area of radiology for your exam, the nurse or technologist will tell you what exam will be performed. In general the electronic ordering process eliminates the errors involved in written, paper-based requests. In addition, all along the way, radiology staff members will verify your identity by checking your wristband and by asking you directly. However, if you feel that you are not in the right area, or are concerned that the exam about to begin is not what you had expected; you should let the technologist or nurse know immediately. There is never harm in asking when in doubt. Occasionally, the Radiologist, in concert with your doctor on the floor, will change or alter the exam in a way that will better address your particular issues. If that is the case, the Radiologist can explain the reason for that change to you. Never let an exam begin if you are not confident that it is correct.

When do I need blood tests checked before I have a Radiology exam?

Blood tests that reflect kidney function will sometimes be checked before a Radiology exam that involves an injection of contrast material. Contrast materials are routinely injected into the vein through an intravenous (IV) line for CT and MRI exams. They are injected through the artery for a catheter angiogram. The contrast agent mixes in with the blood and does exactly what it advertises: as it accumulates in various tissues, it increases the visualized contrast between various tissues in the body, making abnormalities stand out in an obvious way. The term used for contrast accumulation is "enhance". If your kidney function is normal, the contrast will not be a problem. If your kidney function is very abnormal, the radiologist may decide not to inject contrast, may change the type of contrast that is used, or may decide it is best to get a different Radiology exam altogether. If you do have kidney disease, you may receive an IV saline solution before and occasionally after the injection to protect your kidneys.

Should the Radiologist look at my previous studies to see if there are any changes?

Yes they should and they will! Comparison of a current Radiology exam to a prior exam is a basic standard of practice. Since Radiology exams are images, they are showing only one point in time. Imagine how important it is for your doctor to know if the spot on the lung has been there for 5 years and has not changed or if it was not there one year ago and is new. The significance of a fully electronic Radiology Department is that the prior studies performed at that institution will automatically be available to the Radiologist on his workstation, and there is no need to search for them.

Should I bring copies of other studies performed at a different hospital or office with me to the Radiology Department?

You should bring your prior studies either on films or computer disks if appropriate, with you if they are pertinent. Obviously, it would not be necessary to bring films of your old wrist fracture when you come in to the Emergency Room for abdominal pain. So just use common sense. As we said in the previous paragraph, having that second "point in time" for comparison is so important: it may point to the correct diagnosis, eliminate the need to get additional follow-up tests, or even eliminate the need for a biopsy.

If you do have previous studies with you, you should give them to the technologist performing your test. The technologist will then give them to the radiologist. If your study is complicated, such as a CT or an MRI, the Radiologist will hold on to the study until they have finished interpreting and reporting your test.

After handing over such important information, you should be wondering how you are going to get it back, since you may need it in the future. If the exam was an x-ray or mammogram on film that was not "digital", please decide how you want those handled. "Digital" images are stored in their original form electronically and can always be retrieved if the film is lost. Studies given to you on a CD-ROM are by definition, digital. X-ray film that was not "digital" cannot be stored in its original form, and cannot be retrieved. This type of imaging is phasing out, but is still used at many institutions. If you have an original copy be sure you ask for it back.

Prior studies of any sort can be returned directly to you, given to your doctor, or if you prefer, can be filed with the Radiology Department. Many institutions now have the ability to scan your old tests and place them in your electronic file.

Can I speak to a Radiologist about my test results?

The best person to give you your test results is your own doctor. That is the person who knows your medical history as well as a bit about your personality and your sensitivities. Your doctor will be able to place the results of the Radiology test in proper context. An important exception to this is certain type of mammography called "diagnostic mammography", where the Radiologist will give you your results before you leave.

If after speaking to your doctor you find that you still need more information that they cannot give you, then you can and should ask to speak to the radiologist. You can have your doctor contact the radiologist who supervised and interpreted your study, or you can contact the Radiology Administration of the hospital and ask to speak to the Chair or Vice-Chair of the department.

How do I know if the quality of my study was good?

Image quality is continually evaluated during a Radiology exam. Technical parameters are adjusted throughout your exam to make your study as good as possible, preferably excellent. The technologist will not submit an exam that is less than optimal unless it is physically impossible. You can be confident that once the technologist sends you on your way, your exam quality is at the very least, good. Your technologist will be happy to tell you about the image quality, so feel free to ask.

Can I see a copy of my test results?

Absolutely. You can ask your doctor to print you out a copy of your Radiology report. Alternatively, you may request a copy of your report from the Radiology File Room in person, or the File Room can mail a copy to your home. The file room is not allowed to fax the report or send it to an address other than your home to protect your privacy rights.

Can I get a copy of my films?

Absolutely. Most hospital Radiology departments are fully digital and will be happy to give you a copy of your Radiology study on a CD-ROM, generally for a small fee. It is possible to have your exam printed on film, but the cost of x-ray film is much higher because of its silver content. Film is cumbersome and heavy and we advise against it. A CD is much easier to carry around.

How long should I wait before hearing back from my doctor about my studies?

All Radiology departments strive for a 24-hour turn around between the time your exam is completed to the time the report is ready for viewing. Inpatient reports will have a shorter turn around time than that. If your exam was emergent or urgent, the radiologist will call your doctor with the test results soon after it is completed, no matter what time of day or night.

Having a Baby

Arnold J. Friedman, M.D.

Childbirth is a natural process often fraught with danger, that has become dramatically safer over the past hundred years largely due to advances in obstetrics. Improvements in obstetrical care over this time arguably have had more positive impact on outcomes for mothers and their babies than those of any other medical specialty.

The vast majority of pregnancies are normal and require routine prenatal care. The focus of care in these pregnancies is education about the process, screening for abnormalities or risk factors and preparation for delivery and new parenthood. At the other end of the spectrum are the complicated pregnancies. Whether these problems predate pregnancy or develop over the course of pregnancy, they can be extremely dangerous to mother and baby, even life-threatening on occasion. Identification of risk factors before and during pregnancy and the ability to handle complications when they occur are the keys to successful outcomes in these difficult cases.

The best caregivers and hospitals have the ability to provide the full spectrum of obstetrical care tailored to meet the needs of the individual pregnant woman. They don't over treat the normal pregnancy, yet they are ready and able to handle the most difficult problem pregnancies and emergencies.

What should I look for when I choose a doctor or midwife to deliver my baby?

In selecting an obstetrical caregiver it is important above all else to find someone who is well trained, thorough and highly competent. Since most obstetricians and nurse midwives today practice in groups, it is important to have an idea of the qualifications of the other providers in the group as well, since it is very possible one of the others may care for you in labor. The obstetrician or midwife should be certified by the appropriate board or in the process of achieving such certification. He or she should inspire confidence and should be a good listener as well as willing and able to spend time answering questions. His or her office should be responsive and return calls promptly.

In the case of a certified nurse midwife, she should work closely with a competent obstetrician who is immediately available should complications arise. Communication between them should be open and frequent. Since nurse midwives may only take care of normal pregnancies, you should discuss the kinds of complications that would lead to transfer to the obstetrician's care and how you will be screened for such problems as the pregnancy progresses. Ideally, these criteria for transfer should be spelled out clearly in written form between nurse midwife and physician.

What should I look for in choosing the hospital where I plan to deliver?

The general concept in choosing a hospital is similar to choosing a doctor or nurse midwife. The hospital should be capable of providing the full range of obstetrical care from the lowest risk normal pregnancy through the most complicated high risk pregnancy, and should be able to adjust the level of care to the needs of the patient. The best obstetrical hospitals provide twenty-four hour in-house anesthesiologists immediately available to the delivery floor, maternal-fetal medicine experts (perinatologists) to consult on high risk pregnancies, and the highest level neonatal intensive care unit (NICU). These "Level 3" nurseries are staffed by attending neonatology physicians, nurse practitioners and specialist nurses to provide the highly specialized care required by the most critically ill newborns.

Most hospitals provide tours of the obstetrical service to prospective patients. The tour provides a chance to check out the facility, both in terms of the physical plant and the general atmosphere of the delivery floor and postpartum unit. It is an opportunity to see the staff in action. You should get a sense of the staff. Do they appear warm and caring? Do they speak respectfully to one another? Do they seem happy in their work? Is the environment clean and pleasant?

The tour is an opportunity to ask questions. It is worthwhile to ask about the percentage of women using epidural anesthesia, the percent breastfeeding and the availability of breastfeeding support, the number of women or babies requiring transfer to another hospital to deal with complications, the hospital's cesarean section rate, and the level of nursery and availability of anesthesia care. As much as the answers to these and other questions will provide useful information to make your decision, you will also develop a feeling about the place that may be equally valuable.

Should I be concerned if my doctor is not available when it comes time for me to deliver?

The day of the solo practitioner obstetrician has nearly passed. Nowadays the majority of obstetricians and midwives work in groups. Even the remaining lone physicians have coverage arrangements with other doctors.

On the surface, the idea of selecting one provider who will be there for you throughout your whole pregnancy, labor and delivery seems like a good one. But this is unrealistic and in fact potentially dangerous. There is much research about the negative impact of fatigue on performance, suggesting that you are much better off with a fresh obstetrician than one who has been up delivering babies three nights in a row. So in selecting your doctor, take the time to find out about the others in the group and their qualifications. Learn who they are, and even ask to meet them for some of your prenatal visits, just in case one of them is on call when you are in labor.

How do I know if it's safe to have a nurse midwife care for my pregnancy?

Midwifery care is safe and appropriate if you have a normal uncomplicated pregnancy and no medical problems. One should always enter midwifery care with high hopes and expectations for normalcy, but a realistic understanding that this is not always the case. The nine months of pregnancy is a time of many changes during which a seemingly normal pregnancy can become high risk. This is why it is so important that the nurse midwife have a close professional relationship with an obstetrician who can quickly intervene if necessary. Remember, the primary goal is always a healthy mother and baby, but the route to that goal may change along the way.

How do I know when it's safe to request more pain medication during labor?

Unfortunately, labor is a painful process. As a result, modern obstetrical care includes a variety of safe and effective techniques for pain management. These range from behavioral techniques to medications and anesthetic procedures. The most commonly used and effective method today is epidural anesthesia, used by a large majority of women in labor. Obstetricians, nursing staff and of course anesthesiologists have a vast experience in labor pain management, and much research has gone into making it extremely safe. Remember that your caregivers have the same goals you do: to get you through labor and delivery as comfortably as possible with a safe delivery and a healthy mother and baby. So if you need pain relief in labor, ask for it. If there is any reason not to medicate you, your doctor will explain.

If my labor is lasting a long time what questions should I be asking my nurses and doctor?

A good labor team should explain the situation continually. They should volunteer information. But feel free to question them. Ask about whether things are going normally, what you can have for pain, whether progress is appropriate, how the decision for c-section is made.

Can my partner stay with me the whole time while I deliver?

In most hospitals today, as long as things are going well your partner may remain with you throughout labor and delivery, even if cesarean delivery is needed. The only exceptions are if you require general anesthesia or rarely, if you are in an emergency situation in which there is no time to include your partner.

Can my baby stay with me in my room the whole time?

This is called rooming-in. Most hospitals will allow and even encourage this if all is normal. Rooming-in is good for bonding, breast feeding, and helping you experience the needs of your baby in an environment where experienced nurses are available to help. Occasionally a baby may need closer observation requiring transfer to the nursery. When this occurs, parents are generally encouraged to spend as much time as they like with the baby.

How do I know that my baby won't get mixed up with another baby?

All babies are identified and paired with the mother in the delivery room. Both mother and baby are labeled with matching name tags in the form of wrist and ankle bands, either printed or electronically coded. You and your partner should not allow the baby to be taken from you until you confirm these identification bracelets are in place. In addition, all hospitals delivering babies have security systems in place to prevent the rare occurrence of infant abduction. Blood typing and DNA testing are available in the extremely rare circumstance when identity may be in question.

When does my baby need to be in the NICU?

Babies born prematurely or with particular medical problems may require the services of the neonatal intensive care unit (NICU). This unit is staffed by experts in the care of these newborns, including neonatologists, neonatal nurse practitioners and newborn intensive care nursing personnel. It is fairly common for newborns born in difficult circumstances or to mothers with certain medical problems or babies who simply require closer than usual observation to be taken to the NICU for a period of time. In this setting, these babies will receive the closest observation and state of the art treatments that will help them through the transition from intrauterine to independent life. If your baby requires such care, you will be encouraged to spend as much time in the unit as possible. The NICU staff is generally very understanding of your concerns and excellent at explaining your baby's condition and treatment, so feel free to ask questions.

In summary, having a baby is an exciting experience. Modern obstetrics has made tremendous strides to make childbirth safer, less painful and more successful. The informed woman is best able to make decisions on which physician or nurse midwife and which hospital are best for her. Appropriate expectations, good choices and flexibility will go a long way toward achieving the results we all desire: a healthy mother and bab

Surgical Care

Having Safe Surgery

I. Michael Leitman, M.D.

I remember being very apprehensive before my surgery. Even though I am a surgeon and had performed nearly 8,000 operations, I was terrified with the prospect of undergoing anesthesia and an invasive procedure. The simple fact is that millions of people in the United States have uncomplicated surgery each year. And, while I eventually convinced myself of this knowledge, I approached this new experience entirely as a patient. I am glad to say, now that it is behind me, that it was not bad at all.

I hope that the following will allow you to be a better-informed and prepared patient and health care consumer.

How do I choose my surgeon?

Ask around. The best source of information is probably your personal physician. However, don't stop there. Perhaps you know a friend who has had a similar operation or maybe you even know a few doctors. You will feel even more confident in your choice if it is confirmed by someone you know and trust. You might even contact your medical insurance company. Often they have information about surgeons on their panel that have a reputation of quality in performing the procedure that you need.

Be careful. Surfing the Internet, looking at the Yellow Pages and advertisements may not be the best way to select a surgeon. In medicine today, the simple truth is that the busiest surgeons do not need to market themselves through these mediums. Colleagues and patients trust them, and their excellent reputation usually translates into a busy practice. Surfing the Web might give you some interesting medical information but it might not be as reliable as a published source.

Consider getting a second opinion. It is often a good way to ensure that having the operation is the best choice for you. Some health insurance plans may require you to get a second opinion before they agree to pay for certain operations. If your plan does not require this, you may still want to have one. If you are expecting your insurance company to pay for a second opinion, be sure to ask before you get the second opinion. If you get another opinion, be sure to take your records from your first doctor so that you may not have to retake some of the tests. It is also helpful to keep a copy of all of these reports for yourself.

What should I ask my surgeon?

Ask a lot of questions. Being well-informed will make you more knowledgeable and help you to make the best choices. Your surgeon should explain things in a way that you can clearly understand. The more prepared you are at the time of your office visit, the easier it will be to understand your surgeon's explanation. Your surgeon may draw a picture explaining the steps involved in the surgery and provide you with a balanced discussion of the risks, benefits and alternatives—including not having any surgery at all.

Ask if there is more than one way to perform the procedure. One way may require more extensive surgery than another. Ask your surgeon why he or she has chosen one way over another. It may be a matter of preference or due to specific medical decision-making.

Up to 80% of patients forget what their surgeon tells them as soon as they leave the office. Nearly 50% of what they do remember is recalled incorrectly.[1] Be sure take notes. It is also very helpful to bring a family member or a friend with you at the time of the consultation.

It is okay to ask about your surgeon's experience with a particular operation. The number of similar surgeries that your surgeon has performed and performs yearly will give you some measure of their familiarity with your condition. Don't be afraid to ask about their statistics and success rate.

How do I decide about anesthesia and select my anesthesiologist?

Your surgeon or the hospital will likely select your anesthesiologist but if you know of one from someone's prior experience it is all right to let your surgeon or the hospital know your preference. It is likely that your anesthesiologist will be assigned to you just before your operation. Your surgeon and anesthesiologist will discuss your condition and your anesthesiologist will also evaluate your medical history. They will present the options to you before you enter the operating room.

---

[1] Kessels R, Patients' memory for medical information. Journal of the Royal Society of Medicine 2003:96:219-222.

Although there may be a choice of the type of anesthesia, often your surgeon and anesthesiologist will plan this for you—based upon the type of procedure, your general health and making you as comfortable possible. Anesthesia is used so that surgery can be performed without unnecessary pain. Your surgeon can tell you whether the operation is usually done with local, regional, or general anesthesia, and why this form of anesthesia is recommended for your procedure.

- Local anesthesia numbs only a part of your body for a short period of time (similar to a visit to your dentist's office and having a cavity filled). Not all procedures done with local anesthesia are totally pain-free.
- Regional anesthesia numbs a larger portion of your body, for example, the lower part of your body for a few hours. In most cases, you will be awake with regional anesthesia.
- General anesthesia numbs your entire body for the entire time of the surgery. You will be asleep, or unconscious, if you have general anesthesia.

Many people fear general anesthesia. Loss of control, fear of not waking up, or concern about adverse reactions are the top three reservations that patients express. However, many procedures require general anesthesia and it is generally very safe. Death attributable to general anesthesia is said to occur at rates of less than 1:10,000, but these are average figures incorporating both elective and emergency operations with all types of physical conditions.[2]

How do I choose the right place to have surgery?

This is just as important as choosing the right surgeon. Certain hospitals may specialize or have a greater experience in performing specific types of procedures. Additional trained medical personnel and specialized equipment will be available to your surgeon.

Certain Internet sites can be very helpful with providing you with valuable facts that allow you to compare hospitals. Organizations and government agencies are willing to provide you with information that you can trust:

The Joint Commission : *http://www.qualitycheck.org*

Centers for Medicare and Medicaid Services (CMS)
http://www.hospitalcompare.hhs.gov/

---

[2]   Jenkins K, Baker AB. Consent and anesthetic risk. Anesthesia. Oct 2003; 58(10): 962-84.

You surgeon might be on staff at more than one hospital. You may choose a hospital where there are other physicians and specialists that are familiar with your medical history.

The operation may be performed in a few ways:

1. In a hospital as an inpatient (you will be admitted overnight following surgery)
2. In a hospital as an outpatient (someone will be needed to take you home)
3. At an ambulatory surgery center (a facility where surgery is performed but this may or may not be connected to or affiliated with a hospital)
4. In a doctor's office

The operating room has a specialized lighting system that projects a very bright light onto the surgical area. The OR bed is narrow and is designed to permit surgery to be performed in many different positions. The anesthesia machine is located at the head of the bed. This very specialized and highly maintained machine is used to assist in the delivery of anesthesia. Also in this area are other pieces of equipment, such as monitoring devices. As surgical procedures become more complex, specialized professionals use this equipment in administering anesthesia and monitoring/maintaining life functions during surgery.

Who will be present with me during my operation?

.Typically all people present during your operation will have a role to play. The surgeon will often have an assistant (this might be another surgeon, resident or physician's assistant, or registered nurse first assistant). You do not need to worry about your selected surgeon not being there or not performing your operation. Last minute or unannounced substitutions will not occur without your knowledge or consent. The anesthesiologist will be present and may also have a certified registered nurse anesthetist (CRNA) to assist with your care. The operating team also includes a scrub nurse or technician—someone who is also dressed in sterile garments and passes all of the instruments to the surgeon or the assistant(s). A circulating nurse will be present to provide any additional needed materials or equipment during the operation and make notes to document essential aspects of the procedure. One or two observers might be present during your surgery if it is done at a teaching hospital but they are required to introduce themselves to you and request your permission to observe in advance. No one observes your surgery without your knowledge or consent.

What steps do my surgeon and the hospital take to ensure my safety?

Cases of "wrong-site" surgery or "wrong-patient" surgery are exceedingly rare, although when they occur, they certainly do make headlines. The operating room team works very hard to prepare for your operation. Wrong-site surgery—estimated to occur in 1 in 112,994 operations—is prevented by standard protocols[3]. Working in a similar way to a pilot's *pre-flight checklist*, the operating room team uses a number of procedures to avoid these medical errors. One of these is called the "time-out" in which all members of the team review:

1. The patient's identity (with name and another unique identifier)
2. The procedure plan
3. Verification of the proper site of surgery—with the preoperative marking by the surgeon and verification with other documents such as x-rays, reports and even the patient's participation
4. Review of the patient's medication allergies
5. Proper administration of prophylactic antibiotics

Until this time-out is completed to the satisfaction of all members of the surgical team, nothing happens.

Fires in the OR are also very rare. Although electrical and laser equipment is utilized to perform the operation or to keep the patient warm, fires are avoided by preventing such devices from coming in contact with flammable agents. Drills and safety standards are continuously refined to avoid these events.

There has been considerable research on ways to also prevent fatal blood clots (called pulmonary emboli), anesthetic reactions, heart attacks and other dangerous events during or immediately following surgery. All hospitals have protocols or methods to prevent them and these will be implemented during your operation.

Most people have heard of the rare events of a surgical sponge or instrument being left in a body cavity after surgery. In the past, it is estimated that this occurred in less than 1 in 5000 operations (3). While this may require another procedure to remove it, the Operating Room team goes through a very detailed checking and re-checking of all sponges, needles and instruments used. If any member of the team is in doubt, anyone is empowered to order an x-ray before the surgery is completed.

---

[3]   Kwaan M, Studdert DM, Zinner MJ, MD; Gawande AA. Incidence, Patterns, and Prevention of Wrong-Site Surgery. Arch Surg. 2006; 141:353-358.

How do I prepare for the day of surgery?

Make sure that your surgeon and anesthesiologist are aware of all medications that you take (prescription, nonprescription and even herbal). Your physician or their designee will review your medications and instruct you on which ones to take prior to the operation. It is best if you do not smoke or drink alcoholic beverages for at least 24 hours prior to your surgery. Smoking and drinking may increase the time it takes for you to recover from the anesthesia and may prolong the healing process.

Most patients are asked to fast at least 6 hours prior to surgery. This is done to enhance the safety of the anesthesia and to prevent vomiting and aspiration.

When you check into the hospital, much of your medical and registration information will already be there. You will also be checked to make sure that there have not been any interim changes in your health and the members of your surgical team will meet you and ask you questions to become familiar with your condition. Don't be surprised or put-off if they ask you certain questions more than once. Certain things are important to check more than once.

How will my pain be managed?

From the moment that you arrive in the operating room until well after you have been discharged, every effort is made to prevent and control any discomfort that you might experience. Pain is temporary and if you question people who have had recent surgery, most will tell you that it was minimal or that they had no pain at all. Various medications, both short and long-acting, are administered and prescribed by your surgeon and anesthesiologist. When taken as directed, the risk of side effects or dependence is exceedingly low.

While one may not consider any operation to be "routine," technology has evolved to the point where surgery has become safe and effective.

What should I ask my surgeon after the operation?

More than likely, your surgeon will carefully discuss all of the findings observed during the surgery and the details of the operation. This may not occur in the recovery room since you are still recovering from the effects of anesthesia and additional tests may need to be run. You will likely receive discharge instructions for when you should return to the office, what you might experience during recovery, what medications you should be taking (both which of regular medications you should continue and additional ones prescribed to assist you in your recovery), what you should and should not do, when you may return to work or school, drive, your diet, and what to watch out for. There are some additional questions that you should consider asking during your first visit afterwards:

1. Was my surgery successful?
2. Were you able to perform the operation in the way in which you planned?
3. Was there anything about the operation that you had concerns about?
4. When and how will you get the results of any tests run on specimens obtained during the procedure?
5. Will I need any additional treatment or further surgery for my condition?
6. Do you anticipate anything that might complicate my recovery?

Understanding Your Surgery

Martin S. Karpeh Jr., M.D.

Greater than 25 million operations are performed each year in the United States. With few exceptions these procedures are associated with excellent outcomes but the probability of success following surgery is clearly increased when you have knowledge of what to expect. One of the key aspects to having a safe and successful operation is to communicate with your surgeon and anesthesiologist[1]. The give and take of information about you and your procedure will go a long way to ensure that your operation is as safe as it can be. Open communication is vital to creating and maintaining a safe operative experience.[2] The information in this chapter is meant to help guide you to become one of the millions that are successfully treated by surgery each year.

What do I need to know about my surgery?

Understanding the procedure that you are about to have is essential to best prepare yourself for a successful operation. Surgical procedures vary in length, complexity and in the impact on your body. Preparation can be as simple as not eating or drinking after midnight the night before surgery or as complex as taking laxatives and consuming only clear liquids for a day or two before surgery. Discussing the details of your surgery with your surgeon should be the first step in your preparation. Certain operations carry a greater risk of postoperative complications. The risk of getting pneumonia, developing a blood clot or acquiring a wound infection varies with the length and type of operation. Stopping or significantly reducing your smoking if you are a smoker can help reduce your risk for pneumonia following surgery. Certain medications can increase your risk of bleeding during and after surgery. Having a list of all your medications, including vitamins and health food supplements is extremely helpful in identifying products that may cause trouble during surgery. Sharing information about any allergies that you may have, especially to medications or a food is also very important. You can take an active roll in preparing for a successful operation. The national Library of Medicine has an online module on this subject which serves a useful reference if you want to learn more about preparing for surgery. *http://www.nlm.nih.gov/medlineplus/tutorials/ preparingforsurgery/htm/index.htm*

What is a proper informed consent?

A proper informed consent refers to a process in which you get an opportunity to discuss the risks and benefits of a procedure with the surgeon performing that procedure before the procedure is done. The goal of this process is to give you an appreciation of the risks, benefits and consequences of having the operation under consideration. It also allows you to participate in making choices about your care. The consent form is a legal document indicating that you have had an opportunity to discuss your operation with your surgeon and that you understand the risks and benefits of the procedure. The surgeon will ask you to sign this document before surgery. You should not sign unless you are comfortable that you understand what was explained to you about the procedure you are about to have. If you give consent to a procedure but change your mind prior to the operation, you have the opportunity to discuss the procedure again with your surgeon and sign a different consent. This process allows you to express you thoughts and concerns about any and all aspects of the operation that you may have.

A lot has been written about informed consent and if you want to learn more about this process you might find this website helpful:

http://www.emedicinehealth.com/informed_consent/article_em.htm

What questions should I ask my doctor?

It is often difficult to know where to start when faced with having to undergo an operation. When choosing a general surgeon the challenge can be particularly daunting since "General Surgery" covers such a wide range of operative procedures. These procedures vary a great deal in their level of difficulty and in the frequency with which they are performed. Identifying the right surgeon for you can be a challenge yet it is an essential component of having a successful operation. The American College of Surgeons recommends that you use the following two criteria:

1.) The American Board of Surgery offers certification in General Surgery, Vascular Surgery, Pediatric Surgery Surgical Critical Care and Hand Surgery. To become board certified in General Surgery your surgeon is required to pass a written qualifying examination and an oral certifying examination. Therefore the first question to ask is whether your surgeon is certified by the American Board of Surgery. Board certification indicates that your surgeon has successfully completed an approved surgical training program and has demonstrated an acceptable basic level of knowledge in that specialty.

2.) Membership in the American College of Surgeons. The letters FACS after a surgeons name stand for Fellow of the American College of Surgeons. In addition to being certified by the American Board of Surgery it indicates that the individual has submitted to a process to obtain voluntary credential and performance evaluation by their peers. The College keeps a database of it members that is open to the public. If you are interested looking for a Fellow of the College in your area or you want to enquire about an individual surgeon please visit the college website at: *http://web2.facs.org/acsdir/default_public.cfm*

Board certification does not necessarily indicate experience in the particular procedure that you are considering. The best surgeons are those who can combine skill with experience. Once you have identified qualified surgeons you will want to choose a surgeon who has demonstrated experience in the procedure you are about to have. Many surgeons take additional training after completing their residency to do a Fellowship. This gives them added training and experience in areas such as, Minimally invasive surgery, Vascular surgery, and Pediatric surgery or Surgical Oncology to name a few. Inquiring about additional fellowship training will help in choosing a surgeon.

Not all surgeons gain their experience doing fellowships; experience can be obtained over time from particular practice patterns and from working with a more experienced partner. In the later situation your primary doctor can often be very helpful in choosing your surgeon.

The completion of a successful operation requires close follow-up even after you have left the hospital. It maybe important that you continue to see your surgeon for some period of time after surgery, depending on the complexity of the operation, until he or she feels it is safe to resume normal activity. In spite of good preparation and careful technique complications can occur following any operation. Establishing a level of trust is an important aspect of making your final choice in a surgeon.

Can I expect to see my surgeon before my surgery?

You can expect to see your surgeon before surgery. The surgeon will often see you in the area just outside of the operating room known as the holding area before you actually enter the OR suite. This is a good time to confirm the nature of your operation. In situations where you are having surgery on a particular side of your body the surgeon will want to confirm and mark the site where the operation will be performed. Once you have indicated that you had spoken to your surgeon and that you understand what procedure you are having and that all your questions have been answered the anesthesiologist will proceed to prepare you for sleep.

How do I know if my doctor is going to be the one that is performing the surgery?

Simply ask your surgeon if he or she will be performing your operation. The surgeon will not be offended or put off by this question. At Beth Israel Medical Center we do train surgical residents to become board certified surgeons. However, you can be sure that your surgeon will be doing your surgery. The conduct of the surgery and the decisions made are all under the direction of an attending surgeon. Questions have been raised concerning the experience level of a surgical trainee and its impact on patient safety and their outcome. A group of Canadian investigators reviewed nearly 3000 open heart operations (Coronary Artery Bypass Graft procedures) and compared those performed primarily by residents, fellows or attending surgeons[3]. They found no differences between the groups in postoperative complications or deaths, concluding that with appropriate supervision trainees of all levels can be taught safely.

The complexity of some operative procedures does require the assistance of one or more surgeons. In some instances another board certified surgeon may assist in which case your surgeon will perform major aspects of the operation. Having a number of qualified surgeons available for assistance in major hospitals like Beth Israel Medical Center, is a comfort to your surgeon and the entire operative team. Following your operation your surgeon will dictate an operative note describing the procedure and the operative findings. This is a required document for your medical record that indicates what surgeons where involved and their role.

Should my family expect to see my surgeon right after surgery to see how I did?

It is essential that your family members or your designee be kept informed as to how you are doing during and immediately after surgery. You can expect that your family will either meet and/or speak to your surgeon after the operation to receive a report as to your status and the operative findings. It is not uncommon in situations where the operation is lengthy that a family member will get an update from the operating room providing information regarding the progress of your surgery. We understand the anxiety of waiting to hear what is happening during the operation and that is why every effort is made to keep your family informed.

Reference List

1. Zohar E, Noga Y, Davidson E, Kantor M, Fredman B. Perioperative patient safety: correct patient, correct surgery, correct side—a multifaceted, cross-organizational, interventional study. Anesth Analg 2007; 105(2):443-447.
2. Altman DE, Clancy C, Blendon RJ. Improving patient safety—five years after the IOM report. N Engl J Med 2004; 351(20):2041-2043.
3. Guo LR, Chu MW, Tong MZ et al. Does the trainee's level of experience impact on patient safety and clinical outcomes in coronary artery bypass surgery? J Card Surg 2008; 23(1):1-5.

Safe Care After Surgery

David Seres, M.D.

What are my doctors looking for when I am recovering from surgery in the hospital?

Hospitalization after surgery is generally required to fulfill two goals. The first is to provide care that you require due to the surgery and which you would not be able to safely receive at home. This may include such things as simple as frequent dressing changes and antibiotics. It may also include things as complex as mechanical ventilation, balancing of fluid and salt changes, and sophisticated pain management strategies.

The second reason for you to stay in the hospital after surgery is so your team can watch for any signs or symptoms which may indicate a problem. The period of time you spend in the hospital is determined by both how well you are recovering and the odds that a serious complication will occur within a certain time period after your particular surgery.

Your doctors are watching your vital signs (blood pressure, pulse, temperature, breathing rate, oxygen levels, urine output, and pain level) and blood tests to confirm that there is no infection, that there is proper balancing of fluid and salts, and that all of your vital organs (particularly the kidneys, lungs, and liver) are functioning properly. They are checking your surgical wound to make sure it is healing properly, and that there is no break-down, infection or bleeding.

When is it important to tell my doctor or nurse about a problem I am having?

It is never wrong to question something you feel isn't right. You should never allow yourself to be uncomfortable. If your pain is not adequately controlled it may be a sign of a problem. And the experience of pain itself may cause problems. Even if it is a normal amount of pain for the procedure (and some surgery is very painful afterwards), you should make your caregivers aware. Your pain should also decrease by about half each day. If it does not, or it increases, this may signal a problem.

Research has shown that experiencing more pain after surgery may negatively effect healing and your immune system. So avoid the "grin and bear it" approach. And research has also shown that it is extremely unlikely for you to become addicted to pain medicine when it is used after surgery. (see "Pain in the Hospital" section)

After abdominal or chest surgery, severe pain may make it difficult for you to take normal deep breaths or for you to sigh. This in turn increases the risk for pneumonia. You have surely heard someone say: "Don't go to the hospital, you'll get pneumonia." It is not the bad bugs in the hospital that increase your risk of pneumonia. It is lying in bed and not taking deep breaths that increase your risk. Deep breathing and sighs help open lung segments that collapse on an ongoing basis, and minimize the risk for developing pneumonia.

You should also report any other symptom that is unfamiliar to you. In particular, your team needs to know immediately if you have shortness of breath or difficulty breathing, or pain in your chest. These could signal that you have received too much fluid or are having problems with your heart. With careful screening before surgery, heart problems are unusual afterward. But it's better to be safe than sorry.

Is what I am fed after surgery important to my recovery?

Depending on the type of surgery you have, there may be a significant reason to adhere to a particular diet. People who may develop problems swallowing do better with certain textures of food. People who have had surgery on their intestine or are on certain medications may do better with more (or less) fiber, fat, green vegetables, and so on. Your surgical team and the clinical nutritionist should provide you with information about what diet you should follow both on a day-to-day basis as you recover, and before you go home.

It is important that you do not allow yourself to be undernourished for any length of time after surgery. In general, unless you are instructed otherwise, moderation is a good policy. It is okay to follow cravings within reason. It is often easier to eat many smaller snacks throughout the day than it is to eat three normal-sized meals. If you are finding it hard to maintain your usual intake, it is perfectly acceptable to throw out some of the rules and eat high calorie foods (ice cream, pudding, etc.) to make up the difference. However, if you are diabetic, please check with your medical doctor before indulging. Supplements (Ensure®, Boost®, etc) are a good alternative if you aren't able to eat. These can be mixed with flavoring or with fruit in a blender if the taste does not appeal to you.

There is evidence that having food in your intestine very soon after a variety of types of surgery decreases the risk of complications. Even though this may be counterintuitive, this even includes intestinal surgery requiring removal of parts of the intestine. You may need a temporary feeding tube so that your surgeon may accomplish this. This is not the same situation as having a feeding tube inserted at the end of life. Please discuss this with your surgeon in advance of any major intestinal, head and neck, chest, or pelvic surgery.

What other ways can I help with my post-operative recovery?

Most doctors agree that a well-educated patient does best. Read any of the materials your doctor may give you in advance of your surgery. Many conditions that require surgery have support groups and credible websites which may be helpful. Ask your surgeon to help you find them. Make sure that any family members you may have involved in your care educate themselves as well.

Be sure you take advantage of any opportunity to increase your physical activity before and after surgery. As described above, bed rest increases your risk for pneumonia. But bed rest also causes muscle to atrophy and causes a loss of stamina. These may lead to weakness so profound that you might lose the ability to function independently, and your healing may be delayed as well. Even if it is uncomfortable, cooperate with your team when they push you to get out of bed and sit or walk.

Ambulatory Surgery

Donald M. Kastenbaum, M.D.

How do I know if it is appropriate to have my Surgery as Ambulatory Surgery ("Outpatient") or if I need to stay in the hospital?

Your surgeon will answer this for you. Each year in the United States, more and more procedures are being performed as "Outpatient" or Ambulatory procedures. With constant advancements in surgical techniques including: minimally invasive procedures, state of the art equipment, and more advanced anesthetic methods, patients can safely have surgical procedures and recover at home.

I am an Orthopedic surgeon specializing in hip and knee surgery. Occasionally, I may have a case that only requires a "simple" knee procedure; however, a patient might have a specific history or condition such as being "a little older" and/or having recently undergone cardiac bypass surgery six months prior. In cases such as these, I will tell the patient that we will monitor him/her postoperatively, and then make a decision as to whether to let them go home or admit them overnight. In very few instances, a patient may experience more pain than usual and your surgeon may want to admit a patient overnight in order to give stronger pain medication than could be administered at home. Further, a surgeon/primary care physician may want to monitor a patient post-operatively overnight for a pre-existing medical condition.

Remember, each patient's case and circumstances for undergoing surgery is different. Your surgeon will suggest the safest manner for *you* to have an easy and speedy recovery.

What kind of monitoring will I have during my procedure?

Whether you are having Ambulatory Surgery ("Outpatient") or staying in the hospital overnight ("Inpatient"), you will have the same type of monitoring preoperatively (before surgery), intraoperatively (during surgery), and postoperatively (after surgery).

Your surgeon and your anesthesiologist will review your medical history and scheduled procedure, and suggest the best type of anesthesia for you. Remember, your safety and comfort are their most important considerations.

There are several choices for anesthesia including but not limited to combinations of:

- Local anesthesia.
- Regional anesthesia.
- General anesthesia.

For instance, if you were a patient having a knee arthroscopy, you could choose to be wide-awake, while having your knee injected with "numbing medication" (local anesthesia) or a type of regional anesthesia (such as spinal/epidural anesthesia) which numbs a part of your body. However, many patients may *not* want to be awake during the procedure and opt for general anesthesia which numbs the entire body ("being asleep"). Even if you are having local or regional anesthesia, your anesthesiologist can also give you a sedative through your IV to relax you prior to and during your surgery.

Patients worry a great deal about "Anesthesia"—"**Don't**". With proper understanding of the patient's medical history/condition anesthesia is safe. You will meet your anesthesiologist prior to surgery where he/she will review all of this for you. Do not be afraid to tell your anesthesiologist your worries/concerns and make an informed decision about the kind of anesthesia you will have.

What do I look for when I am selecting a facility for my Ambulatory Surgery?

You have already chosen your surgeon. He/she may work at more than one hospital and/or Ambulatory Surgery Center. Ambulatory Surgery Centers are State approved facilities that have their own credentialing process, which in most instances is different from the credentialing process in a hospital. Furthermore, the facilities are free standing, and usually are not affiliated with a hospital, but owned by investors, or even your surgeon.

You should ask your surgeon where he/she usually performs your type of scheduled procedure. You may ask other questions including but not limited to:

- How long has he/she worked there?
- What is the anesthesia and nursing/technical staff like?
- Does he/she benefit financially from you having your procedure there?

If you desire, hospitals and most Ambulatory Surgery Centers will allow you to tour their facilities preoperatively.

Although you have chosen a surgeon you trust, it is your responsibility not to leave any stone unturned—if you have any questions or concerns, Ask! Ask! Ask!

What questions should I ask my doctor when choosing a surgeon? Ask everything!

- Why are you recommending this particular surgeon?
- How many years has this particular surgeon been in practice?
- How many of this type of procedure has this particular surgeon performed?
- How long have you been referring him/her patients?
- Are your patients happy with this particular surgeon's results?
- Do you refer only to one surgeon?
- Can you speak with other patients that have been treated by this surgeon?

Most importantly—do your own homework! If you know about your condition, do research on the internet before you meet your surgeon. Take a list of relevant questions that have arisen from your research when you meet your surgeon. Most patients are "nervous" and "forget" much of what their surgeon tells them—make sure to write down notes and important information. Lastly, upon leaving your surgeon ask "When is the best time to call if you have future questions?"

Patients not only want to know that their surgeons are skilled technicians, but also want surgeons that answer their questions and support their emotional needs/fears. Do not be scared to ask your surgeon *anything*! Remember, there is more than one good surgeon who can treat you . . .

What happens if I develop a complication during my procedure?

There are risks with any surgical procedure. Although most of them rarely occur, if they do your surgeon and the hospital or Ambulatory Surgery Center will deal with them effectively and efficiently. Part of the benefit of having your procedure performed by an experienced surgeon means he/she has "seen it all before" and immediately knows how to respond to all situations. Detailed policies and procedures have been developed to deal with these rare situations. It is worth noting, if you are having surgery at a hospital, it is likely that almost anything your surgeon may need will be at his/her fingertips. On the other hand, if you are having your procedure performed at an Ambulatory Surgery Center, you may need to be transferred to a hospital to get the type of care that is required.

Ask your surgeon, which will be the safest place for *you*.

What do I need to do to prepare for my surgery?

Make checklists for:

- Leading up to surgery—what do I need to do?
- The day of surgery.
- After the operation/recovery.

Leading up to surgery

- What do I need to do?
- Why now?
- Are your expectations realistic?
- Are you physically and emotionally prepared?
- Do you have a support network?
- Have you considered and accepted the risks?
- Do you need to prepare anything at home prior to surgery?
- Do you need any forms filled out by your doctor?
- Did you complete your medical clearance?
- Do you have someone to take you to the hospital?

The day of surgery

- How am I going to get to the hospital/Ambulatory Surgery Center?
- What time do I need to be there?
- Can I bring a book and/or headphones to listen to music?
- Do I have any last minute questions/concerns?
- Do you have someone to take you home after surgery?
- Who is going to fill your prescriptions?
- Can your doctor give you your prescriptions prior to the day of surgery

After the operation

- When is my follow up appointment?
- How long is my recovery?
- How will I know my recovery is going well?
- Is there anything in particular I should watch for?
- Do I have any restrictions?
- When can I drive?
- When can I return to work?

Should I take my medications the morning of surgery?

Medications include: prescription drugs, non-prescription drugs, and herbal remedies.

Should I take my medications the morning of surgery is a question that will have a different answer for each and every patient. When you first meet your surgeon, he/she will note your detailed medical history. This is done to allow your doctor to learn *everything* about your medical health, not only about the specific condition you are meeting with the surgeon about. From my personal experience of having performed more than 6,000 procedures, I know within minutes of meeting a patient which orthopedic treatment will benefit them the most. Yet, I spend a long time discussing medical histories in order to learn about my patients' general health, what procedures they may have previously had, what medications they take, any allergies they might have, and their family history.

So to get back to the answer . . . if you take medications daily, your surgeon and/or your primary care physician will tell you which medications to either not take the day of surgery or which medications to take the day of surgery with a "sip" of water. Your surgeon and/or your primary care physician may also tell you to stop taking some of your medications a week or more prior to surgery. In general, all herbal remedies and aspirin-type medications are stopped a week or more prior to surgery.

Remember, if you have any questions, ask your surgeon!

Can I expect to see my surgeon before my operation?

Absolutely! Most surgeons are very responsive to the needs of their patients and want to speak with them prior to surgery to discuss any final concerns/questions that patients may have.

Furthermore, as of on March 1, 2007, the State of New York Department of Health instituted the New York State Surgical and Invasive Procedure Protocol (NYSSIPP) for hospitals, surgery centers, and individual practitioners. Part of this new set of protocols is that the attending physician/dentist/ podiatrist doing the procedure must mark the surgery site with his/her own initials prior to the patient being taken into the operating room.

Should my family expect to see my surgeon right after surgery?

Yes. After a surgical case is finished, the patient is accompanied to the Post Anesthesia Care Unit (PACU) or better known as the "Recovery Room". I then explain to my patient the operative findings, explain to them what was done during the successful procedure, and what I expect their outcome to be.

A family member or significant other of the patient is then brought into the PACU. If neither a family member nor significant other is able to be there after surgery, have them provide a telephone number where the surgeon can contact him/her to advise of the results of surgery.

Although most surgeons follow the same procedure that I described above, some may not. Just like any interaction with people in life, tell your surgeon "what is important to you". Most surgeons are very accommodating and will make every effort to provide the *ultimate* patient experience for you.

Specialty Services

Cancer Care

Louis Harrison, M.D. and Michael Grossbard, M.D

With so many choices for treating cancer, how do I know which treatment option is best for me?

The diagnosis of cancer is accompanied by significant emotional stress. This is a life-threatening illness, and all decisions must be approached with thoughtfulness and comprehensiveness. As with many diseases, cancer affects the entire family, not just the individual patient. Loved ones come together, work as a team and make major decisions as a family unit. The emotional and intellectual support of loved ones is essential to decision-making, and to achieving the best outcome.

The treatment options for cancer will vary, depending upon many factors:

What part of the body is affected?

A 2 cm. cancer of the colon is dramatically different than a 2 cm. cancer of the breast. The options are different, and the outcomes are different.

What stage is the cancer?

The treatment of any given cancer will differ by its size, whether it has spread to lymph nodes, or whether it has spread to other organs.

What is the exact pathologic type of cancer?

A cancer diagnosis is made by a pathologist who looks at a biopsy specimen under a microscope. The accurate interpretation of this biopsy is essential for proper care. Within each organ of the body, many different types of cancer can arise. For example, in the skin a cancer can be a melanoma, a squamous cell carcinoma, a basal cell carcinoma, or one of many other possibilities. Depending upon the exact type, the treatment options will vary.

Given all of these issues, it is common for a variety of treatment options to be considered for every patient. While it is true that many patients will have one clear option, a large percentage of patients face a variety of options to consider. Many patients will require several treatments. Therefore, in order to make the best decision, cancer patients should seek the advice of multiple specialists. The three main cancer treatments are surgery, radiation therapy, and chemotherapy. Thus, most cancer patients benefit from consultations with a surgeon, a radiation oncologist, and a medical oncologist. It is best when these specialists are working together as a team, usually in the same medical center. This assures that the patient is getting a coordinated approach, and that all options are being considered. The patient should understand the differences between the options, their pros and cons, and relative advantages and disadvantages. It is essential to understand the cure rates that can be obtained with different treatments, as well as the side effects/complications. Some patients will accept a smaller cure rate in order to avoid certain complications such as impotence, disfigurement, or other permanent disabilities. An important concept in current cancer management is "organ and function preservation." Our goal is to treat the cancer while maximizing the functional capabilities of each patient. Nowadays, most women with breast cancer do not need to lose their breast. They can be treated with limited surgery, radiation therapy, and preserve their breast. Patients with tongue cancer, larynx cancer, cancers near the eye, can often be treated with sophisticated radiation therapy or chemotherapy/radiation therapy approaches, avoiding the need to remove these important organs. Today, most patients with rectal cancer can be treated with combinations of surgery, radiation therapy and chemotherapy, which avoid the need for a permanent colostomy. Management strategies for prostate cancer, with innovative radiation therapy and surgical approaches, can minimize complications such as impotence and incontinence. No matter what organ is affected by cancer, the patient should understand whether there are options that maximize the chances of cure as well as organ and function preservation.

With new technology and new methods to combine treatments, there has been a growth of non-invasive and minimally invasive strategies. It is important for every patient to see if they are a candidate for strategies that are the least uncomfortable, will inflict the least disability, and will get them back to a normal and productive life as soon as possible.

Every patient needs to pick the right balance of cure rate and quality of life, in choosing the treatment option that is right for them. Indeed, this could be the biggest decision of anyone's life. Getting all the information, speaking to the appropriate experts, listening to loved ones, are all essential. Once the decision has been made, move forward and never look back.

How do I decide where and with whom to get my care?

Having made the decision about treatment options, the next key choice is where, and with whom to get your care. It is essential to select the best medical environment, and the best people, in order to obtain the best results. No doubt, during the process of deciding treatment options, most patients will encounter multiple physicians, potentially at multiple medical centers. The best outcomes are obtained by expert teams of physicians who are working together in a coordinated way. The team includes specialists in surgical oncology, radiation oncology, medical oncology, pathology, diagnostic imaging, supportive care services, and multiple other areas. Colleagues in nursing, nutrition, psychosocial counseling, complimentary medicine, research, social work, and a myriad of other areas, are also required. It is not unusual for a typical cancer patient to require the expert care and services of dozens of professionals. Thus, in selecting the medical team and medical center for your care, patients should make sure that this type of comprehensive approach will be available to them. It is well-established that the best model for this type of care is the "cancer center." A cancer center brings together all of the experts that are required for the complex and well-coordinated care that every patient requires. Patients should seek this environment for optimal care.

There are nationally-accepted standards that cancer centers must follow in order to receive accreditation by important national organizations such as the National Cancer Institute, the American College of Surgeons—Commission on Cancer, or some other major accrediting body. In order to receive accreditation, cancer centers must be able to provide a wide range of specialists, have the latest technology, participate in clinical trials and other aspects of cancer research. They must diligently keep track of their outcomes, demonstrate that their outcomes are consistent with national and published standards, that they follow accepted standards of care for every type and stage of cancer, and that the cancer specialists meet regularly to discuss cases and review their treatment. Quality measures must be demonstrated that assure the entire spectrum of cancer services are provided in a programmatic framework which optimizes the patients' results. Every patient and family should seek to know that they are being treated in this type of medical environment.

Finally, it is important for patients to be treated in a caring and healing environment. Nowadays, it is not enough to just treat the cancer. Providing personal and family comfort, social work services, emotional support, as well as complimentary/integrative therapies all promote the best possible outcome. Ask about these issues, and learn what is available. The treatment of every patient should be individualized, personal and caring.

How is cancer care coordinated?

As described above, cancer care is a team approach. It is essential for patients to seek counsel from all of the involved cancer specialists. Once a treatment program has been designed, usually multiple cancer specialists will need to coordinate the care in a seamless fashion. For example, a patient with throat cancer might require a combination of radiation therapy and chemotherapy followed by surgery. In this situation, a radiation oncologist, medical oncologist and surgeon will all have to work together to coordinate the care. Not only the physicians, but also the nursing staff and support staff need to work together so that care is seamless. It is most helpful when these specialists are working together in a single center, often in locations near one another. This fosters collaboration, coordination of care and patient convenience. In the best circumstances, the treatment team is so highly coordinated, and communicates on such a regular basis, that the patient sees the entire multi-disciplinary team as a single unit.

How do I know if I should get chemotherapy in the doctor's office or in the hospital?

Chemotherapy refers to the administration of drugs to treat cancer. Most often, these agents are administered intravenously (through the vein), although an increasing number of chemotherapy agents are available in pill form. There are several locations where patients can receive chemotherapy including a doctor's office, the outpatient department of a hospital, a freestanding cancer center, or in the inpatient setting of a hospital.

Some chemotherapy regimens, particularly those that place the patient at high risk of nausea or vomiting, or high risk of acute complications, including allergic reactions, during the time of the treatment, require administration in the hospital. At the present time, relatively few treatment programs with chemotherapy require in-patient hospitalization. The most common chemotherapy drugs administered in the hospital include high-dose Cisplatin and high-dose Methotrexate, both of which require close monitoring and the vigorous administration of intravenous fluids during the course of treatment. Furthermore, some patients require chemotherapy in the hospital particularly if they are too ill to receive safe treatment in the outpatient setting.

Despite the above caveats, the overwhelming majority of chemotherapy is administered in the outpatient setting. Chemotherapy can safely be administered either at a doctor's office, a hospital outpatient department, or a freestanding cancer center. Most importantly, the patient must feel comfortable with the treatment team, skilled nurses are available and appropriate precautions should be taken to ensure the safe administration of chemotherapy and to handle any emergencies that may arise.

Ideally, the patient should have an opportunity to view the treatment area prior to initiating therapy. The area should be clean and have ample space for the patient to sit comfortably during treatment. The patient should be able to verify that the nursing staff has experience with chemotherapy administration. Specifically, the patient can assess whether the training program regarding the risks and toxicities of various chemotherapy agents. For example, oncology nurses should complete a rigorous training course followed by a period of supervision by previously trained oncology nurses before they are permitted to administer chemotherapy to our patients.

Occasionally, emergencies arise with the administration of chemotherapy. For instance, allergic reactions necessitating rapid intervention can occur. Patients should make certain that the facility in which they are treated has a plan in place to address chemotherapy emergencies.

The treating physician and his/her team should be able to explain the reasons why they have chosen to administer chemotherapy at a particular location for a specific patient.

I've heard terrible stories about medical errors. How do I know that everything is being done correctly with dosing my chemotherapy?

Chemotherapy agents have the potential to offer life-saving and survival enhancing treatments to patients with cancer. Unfortunately, these agents also have significant risks. For example, an adequate vein needs to be obtained to administer chemotherapy because some agents can cause severe damage to the skin if they leak (extravasate) from the vein during treatment. Some drugs must be diluted significantly and administered over a slow rate to prevent reactions, including drops in blood pressure and shortness of breath. Other agents can be safely administered through the vein, but if mistakenly administered into another region of the body (such as the spinal fluid), it can cause paralysis and even be lethal. It is incumbent upon the providing team to make sure that proper checks and balances are in place for each patient who receives chemotherapy.

The proper dosing and administration of chemotherapy is critical to safe administration. Several local and national organizations have studied the process of chemotherapy administration and have recommended several checks that should be put in place by those administering chemotherapy to make certain that the proper agents are administered in the proper dose, schedule and location to patients with cancer. A patient with cancer should feel free to question his or her physicians and nurses regarding the procedures in place at their center to insure that chemotherapy is administered with the utmost safety.

At Continuum Cancer Centers of New York, we have written policy guidelines regarding the ordering and administration of chemotherapy. All orders are generated in a computer-based system so that dose calculations are done by the computer rather than by hand, thereby minimizing human error. In addition, the requirement for electronic orders means that there will not be difficulty interpreting handwriting since some chemotherapy agents have similar names but very different uses. The chemotherapy order initially is reviewed by a treating nurse to confirm the patient name, the diagnosis, the treatment regimen, the correct dosing, and to make certain that the patient's blood counts are adequate for treatment. The chemotherapy order is then delivered to the pharmacy where the pharmacist recalculates the patient's dose, reviews prior treatment regimens to make certain that the administered therapy is consistent with the prior dosing and enters the orders into the patient's pharmacy profile. Labels are then printed for each medication to be administered containing cautions and warnings related to the specific drug. The medication is then mixed by the pharmacist just prior to the time of administration. The patient is then identified and the chemotherapy drugs are checked yet again to make certain that the correct treatment is being administered to the correct patient.

What precautions should be taken if I become immunosuppressed due to my medications or my disease?

One of the major risks of chemotherapy is immunosuppression. In many cases, cancer itself can lead to a suppressed immune system either because the disease directly impairs the immune system, or because poor nutritional status contributes to decreased immunity. For example, patients with multiple myeloma, leukemia, and lymphoma often have direct immune system deficits due to the underlying disease process itself. Patients with impaired nutritional status are less able to fight off infection than those patients with adequate nutrition.

Chemotherapy itself can impair the immune system. Many chemotherapy drugs battle cancer by directly killing tumor cells. Unfortunately, this cell death is often not specific and normal cells, including white blood cells that fight infection, can be destroyed along with the tumor cells. Fortunately, this decline in white blood count usually lasts for only a brief period of time before the body again starts to produce a normal white blood count. More severe immunosuppression can be seen in the setting of high dose chemotherapy when patients undergo bone marrow or stem cell transplants.

Many infections that people with cancer and impaired immune systems develop are caused by bacteria that colonize the mouth and gastrointestinal tract in all individuals. Visiting a dentist prior to chemotherapy and maintaining good oral hygiene during the treatment can reduce the risk of infection. The treating physician will decide whether the patient may benefit from the administration of prophylactic antibiotics. Alternatively, some patients receive drugs right after their chemotherapy (filgrastim, perfilgrastim) that can reduce the risk of infection by helping the white blood count to the decline less and recover faster.

Some chemotherapeutic agents can cause neutropenia, a drop in the numbers of a particular type of white cell known as polymorphonuclear leukocytes. When patients become neutropenic, they will be advised to wash their hands well and avoid other individuals who have active communicable infections. Fresh fruits and fresh flowers can be a source of bacteria and it is recommended that neutropenic patients avoid these exposures.

Despite the immunosuppression that accompanies chemotherapy, a relatively small percentage of patients develop significant infections that require hospitalization. Maintaining good contact with the treatment care team and making sure that they are aware of any fevers, mouth sores, or developing illnesses at the earliest possible time is critical to ensuring favorable outcomes. While immunosuppression is a severe and expected complication of chemotherapy, all medical oncologists are trained in its management and should be able to work directly with the patient to minimize risks.

Web Sites

www.ASCO.org	American Society of Clinical Oncology
www.ASTRO.org	American Society for Therapeutic Radiology and Oncology
www.cancercare.org	Cancer Care
www.cancer.org	American Cancer Society
www.cancer.gov	National Cancer Institute
www.gildasclub.org	Gilda's Club
www.canceradvocacy.org	National Coalition for Cancer Survivorship
www.thewellnesscommunity.org	The Wellness Community
www.cancer.net	ASCO Cancer Foundation
www.rtanswers.org	ASTRO Patient Resource site
www.surgonc.org	Society of Surgical Oncology
www.wehealny.org/services/cancer	Continuum Cancer Centers of New York

Having an Endoscopy Procedure

Brett Bernstein, M.D.

How Do I Tell if My Endoscopy Center is High Quality?

Word of mouth and personal experience are the criteria most people use to gauge the quality of the care they receive. Although these are important in making a choice, there are other more objective criteria that can be used to make an educated decision. High quality endoscopy centers should have licensure by the State, certification to participate in Medicare/Medicaid programs, and accreditation by a nationally recognized organization such as The Joint Commission.

Accreditation represents recognition for complying with rigorous national performance standards that focus on the quality and safety of care provided. The process of accreditation is voluntary and involves a detailed on-site survey by health care professionals who examine the center's physical surroundings, interview staff members, and observe how care is delivered.

What Do I Need to Do to Prepare for My Procedure ?

Before your procedure, you will receive detailed instructions from your physician on how to prepare. You should discuss your medical history in detail with your physician, as well as your medications, including anything you might be taking over the counter such as nutritional supplements, cold medicines, or pain relievers. Certain medications such as aspirin and other over the counter painkillers have blood thinning properties and will need to be discontinued prior to your procedure. Let your doctor know if you are taking any of these.

If you are going to have an upper endoscopy, also known as an "EGD", you will need to fast for at least 6 hours prior to your procedure.

If you are going to have a colonoscopy, your preparation will involve taking a laxative preparation on the day prior to your examination. There are a variety of laxative preparations available including liquids, tablets, and combinations of the two. These preparations work by flushing your intestines with fluid and sometimes stimulating contractions of the intestines. Your diet will generally be limited to clear liquids for 24 hours prior to your appointment. It is important to drink adequate amounts of fluid prior to your procedure to avoid dehydration.

Who are the Various Professionals that will be Involved in my Care?

You will have contact with a variety of health care providers prior to, during, and after your procedure. A nurse will usually perform a brief interview prior to your procedure in order to obtain accurate information about your medical history and medications. You should bring an accurate list of your current medications, including the dosage, to your appointment. A set of vital signs will be taken at this time including your blood pressure, pulse rate, and temperature. The nurse may place an intravenous line, which is a small plastic tube, into a vein in your arm at this time. This tube will allow the doctor to administer the medication needed to make you sleepy and comfortable during the procedure. The intravenous line insertion feels like getting stuck by a sewing needle, similar to having blood drawn. In the procedure room, you will meet another nurse who will help prepare you for the procedure and will assist your doctor during the procedure. When your doctor arrives, you should ask any questions you might have at this time. The doctor will have you sign a consent form for your procedure after he or she has discussed the risks, benefits, and alternatives. An anesthesiologist may be present to administer the medication to make you sleepy and comfortable. This doctor may also ask you questions about your medical history and any previous experience with anesthesia. Following the procedure you will be taken to a recovery area where another nurse will monitor you for approximately one hour or until you are stable for discharge.

What type of monitoring should I expect during my procedure?

Before your procedure is performed, a variety of devices will be placed on your body to monitor your vital signs. A blood pressure cuff will be placed around your upper upper arm and will inflate and deflate automatically to take your blood pressure. A probe will be placed on one of your fingers to measure the oxygen level in your blood. Small stickers attached to wires will be place on your chest to monitor your heart rhythm. These devices will remain in place until you have fully recovered and are ready to be discharged.

What type of anesthesia should I expect during my procedure?

The most common type of anesthesia administered for endoscopy and colonoscopy is referred to as moderate sedation. Medication will be administered through an intravenous line that will make you very sleepy, calm, and have no significant memory of the procedure. Unlike general anesthesia which requires your breathing to be supported by a machine called a ventilator, during endoscopic procedures you will be breathing on your own. Prior to an upper endoscopy, the physician may also administer a "topical" anesthetic to the back of your throat in the form of a spray or liquid.

How long will I need to recover from my procedure?

In general, it will take approximately 1 hour to recover from your procedure. However, as some people may feel drowsy for several hours, it is not advisable for you to drive or operate heavy machinery following your procedure. In addition, it is mandatory that you have a friend or family member escort you home following discharge.

What Happens if I develop a Complication During My Procedure?

Endoscopy and colonscopy are very safe procedures and complications occur in less than 1 percent of patients. Some of the complications that can occur include but are not limited to the following:

1. Aspiration of food or fluids into the lungs is rare and the risk can be minimized by fasting for at least 6 hours prior to your examination.
2. The endoscope can rarely cause a perforation, which is a hole or tear. The risk of this occurring is less than 1 out of every 3000 procedures. If this occurred you would need to remain in the hospital for observation and rarely might require an operation.
3. Bleeding is a rare complication that can occur after the removal of polyps or if biopsies are taken. The risk of this occurring is less than 1 out of every 3000 procedures. Most patients stop bleeding spontaneously, but under rare circumstances the doctor may have to perform another endoscopic procedure to stop the bleeding. If the bleeding is still not controlled, an operation may be required.

4. Sometimes, the vein into which the intravenous line has been placed may become irritated. Irritation will be indicated by redness, swelling, or warmth at the site. If this happens you can apply a warm cloth to the site to relieve the discomfort. If discomfort persists, you should call your primary care provider, gastroenterologist, or the endoscopy unit. If this is not possible, you should seek assistance in an emergency department.

Cardiac Catheterization

John T. Fox, MD FACC

A cardiac catheterization is an invasive procedure meaning the skin is penetrated and instruments enter the body. It is used as a secondary means of defining coronary artery disease in patients who have a stable condition. Two major disease categories which are dealt with in the adult cardiac catheterization laboratory are coronary artery disease and valvular heart disease.

What are the indications for a Cardiac Catheterization?

Valvular heart disease is commonly seen in the catheterization laboratory. The heart is a pump with four chambers and four valves. The right side of the heart is a low pressure system that receives blood from the body and then pumps the blood to the lungs. The left heart is a high pressure system which pumps the oxygenated blood it receives from the lungs to the entire body. A valve that leaks (regurgitation) or a valve that does not open fully (stenotic) can lead to heart failure. Pressure measurements are recorded inside the heart. Pictures of the heart chamber (ventriculograms) and pictures of the main blood vessel of the body (aortagrams) can show leaky valves. These pictures and pressure measurements help make the diagnosis and determine the severity of the valve disease.

An echocardiogram (sound pictures of the heart) is a non-invasive test and is the preferred way of diagnosing valvular heart disease. Catheterizations are still used when there are questions about the echocardiogram readings. If surgery is needed to fix the valve, coronary angiograms are performed to diagnosis any coronary artery disease which then can be fixed (grafted) at the same time the valve is fixed. Certain stenotic valvular heart disease can also be treated in the catheterization lab with balloon therapy. Research is now under way to fix and even replace all types of diseased valves in the catheterization lab without the need for surgery.

The vast majority of the patients that come through the cardiac catheterization lab are being evaluated for coronary artery disease. Atherosclerosis is the build-up of cholesterol causing a narrowing of the artery and a decrease in blood flow. This process can happen in any of the arteries of the body and when it occurs in the heart arteries it is called coronary artery disease. The three patterns of coronary artery disease are: the stable plaque, the unstable plaque or an occlusive plaque.

The cholesterol plaque in the stable pattern is older with a thick cap that has a tendency not to rupture but is obstructive to blood flow causing symptoms especially with exertion. The unstable plaque is fast growing and has a thin cap which has ruptured. The blood sees this ruptured plaque as if it was a "cut in the skin" and wants to form a clot to heal it. This clot formation can be harmful because it can close the artery fully and stop blood flow. With an unstable plaque opening and closing of the artery is occurring and the patient is experiencing symptoms. These symptoms can be at rest or occurring with minimal activity lasting minutes in an intermittent pattern. This stage is where drugs can stop the clot formation and prevent a heart attack. If the unstable plaque closes and does not open an occlusive plaque is formed. The blood flow is unable to pass the blockage and heart muscle is injured and then dies (heart attack). Symptoms are at rest, are constant and remain for hours. According to the American Heart Association's annual statistical report, coronary artery disease causes about 1.2 million deaths or heart attacks per year in the United States. [1] The majority of patients have the stable pattern.

RISK FACTORS AND SYMPTOMS

Certain members of the population have a greater chance of having coronary artery disease and there are known risk factors. The classic risk factors are: age, male sex, hyperlipidemia, hypertension, diabetes, family history of premature coronary artery disease (onset of disease <55 male <65 female primary relative), smoking and obesity.

There are also classic symptoms people can get when the coronary artery disease becomes obstructive to blood flow—"Angina Pectoris" which is the classic phrase used to describe chest pain caused by narrowing of the heart arteries actually means "choking in the chest". Thus, the discomfort of angina often is described not as pain, but rather as an unpleasant sensation; "pressing," "squeezing," "strangling," "constricting," "bursting," and "burning" are some of the adjectives commonly used to describe this sensation."[2] This sensation can occur alone, can radiate to the arm or jaw and can be associated with other symptoms such as nausea/vomiting, shortness of breath, fatigue and loss of consciousness (passing out). Some people have no symptoms at all which is known as "silent ischemia".

When symptoms occur or in certain high risk asymptomatic groups evaluation by an internist and referral to a cardiologist should occur. If the symptoms and risk factors put the likelihood of having obstructive coronary artery disease in a medium range a non-invasive work up (stress testing) is often done first. There is newer technology such as Computed Tomography (CT) Angiography and calcium scores which also help determine the likelihood of having coronary artery disease. People with risk factors, typical symptoms and or abnormal stress tests are the majority of patients who present with coronary artery disease in this stable pattern.

People with unstable or occlusive plaques have symptoms at rest, with minimal exertion or with increasing frequency and should go to the emergency room. Medications can be started to prevent the clot formation and an urgent or emergent visit to the catheterization lab can be arranged to diagnose and treat the ruptured plaque or heart attack.

What Happens in the Cath Lab?

The catheterization laboratory is where pictures of the heart arteries are taken. A small tube with a one way valve is inserted into the leg or arm artery. This initial tube allows wires and longer tubes (catheters) to be inserted into the body and reach the heart arteries without bleeding. The arteries do not have nerves so these thin wires and tubes are not felt by the patient. The skin is sensitive to pain and a local anesthetic is used to "numb the skin" prior to the placement of the initial tube. Dye is injected through the long tubes and is directed into the heart artery. An x-ray camera takes moving images of the dye as it flows through the arteries. It shows where the artery is narrowed by the cholesterol plaque. This is the diagnostic part of the procedure and allows decisions to be made on how to manage the patient. The pattern and location of the plaques, the heart function and the overall health of the patient determine which therapeutic options should be rendered. The three options are medical management, cardiac surgery or an intermediate step which is called an "interventional approach".

An interventional cardiologist has special training to take the diagnostic procedure and transform it into a therapeutic procedure. Through the same initial tube placed, a special guiding catheter is advanced to reach the narrowed heart artery. An intervention (opening of the narrowing) can immediately follow the diagnostic portion. Sometimes for clinical reasons, complexity of disease and to review different therapeutic options the intervention is scheduled on another day. The interventional procedure entails placing a thin wire through the guiding catheter into the heart artery and past the blockage. This wire acts as a rail, so devices can be safely guided to the blockage. A balloon catheter with a metal coil (stent) mounted on it is most commonly used. It is delivered to the plaque and the balloon is inflated pressing and implanting the metal coil into the wall of the artery. The balloon is removed and the coil acts as "scaffolding" being incorporated into the wall and opening the narrowed part of the artery. The exposed metal is a place where a clot can form, similar to the ruptured cholesterol plaque. Aspirin and clopidogrel need to be taken for at least one month for an "uncoated" (bare metal) stent to inhibit the platelets (the blood particles which start clot formation). When the stent healing is complete the platelet blocking can be lessened or continued unchanged depending on the state the patient.

What is Restenosis?

The trauma caused by expanding the artery with the stent triggers an inflammation response in the artery. This inflammation leads to tissue growth within the stent. Tissue can form an "overgrown scar" and block the stented area causing a decrease in blood flow again. This process is called restenosis and usually is seen at three to six months peaking at nine months. Some regression of the scar may be seen at nine to twelve months and the majority of the tissue growth is over at one year.

Restenosis can be obstructive causing symptoms to reoccur in approximately fifteen percent of cases (depending on what was treated) and may occasionally lead to a heart attack. If symptoms reoccur or a stress test becomes positive again; it is important to undergo a catheterization to diagnose and treat the restenosis.

Efforts to decrease restenosis led to the development of a coated (drug eluting) stent. The medicine which coats the stent limits the scar formation, so the rate of restenosis is reduced. Multiple randomized clinical trials have demonstrated a reduction in restenosis of up to fifty percent or greater. Drug eluting stents have allowed the treatment of more aggressive patterns of plaque, without the need for open heart surgery.

The downside of blunting restenosis is that a longer amount of time is required to inhibit platelet function so the stent heals without forming a clot in it. Aspirin and clopidogrel should be given for at least one year for coated stents. This is different from the one month needed for uncoated stents. An important point to be made is that whenever aspirin and clopidergol are going to be stopped, the interventional cardiologist or the general cardiologist (who knows the patient well), should be involved in curtailing their use in a safer way.

Will I Need a Stent?

Stents in the stable plaque can relieve symptoms but do not prevent a heart attack or make one live longer. It is similar to plumbing, opening a blocked pipe to increases flow or an artery to increase flow will help take away symptoms. If one does not change what goes down the pipe or artery it will block again in a new spot and cause a heart attack or new symptoms. The real way to prevent the progression of plaque build-up is by lowering one's risk factors. Behavior modification with smoking cessation, low cholesterol diet, regular exercise, reducing stress, controlling blood pressure and blood sugars is critical in preventing future events. Clinical trials have convincingly demonstrated that the cholesterol lowering effects of "statin" medications have decreased subsequent cardiovascular events (preventing new blockages).

Platelet inhibition medications (aspirin and clopidogrel) have played an important role in decreasing heart attacks. They act on the clotting part of the unstable plaque so it can heal without becoming totally closed off and causing a heart attack. These drugs also keep the stent free of clot, until it has a chance to fully heal. Other drugs which control blood pressure, heart rates and dilate the arteries are used to control or lessen symptoms (beta-blocker or nitrates) and some to prevent heart attacks from reoccurring (ace-inhibitors).

In patients who have an unstable plaque or an occlusive plaque, opening the artery with stents can stop the heart attack and improve the person's chances of living through the heart attack.

How Should I Prepare for My Catheterization?

In preparing for an elective or scheduled catheterization, one should not eat after midnight before the procedure. Patients lie flat during the procedure so it is important to have a relatively empty stomach because the contrast dye and sedatives occasionally make patients vomit.

Patients should continue to drink normal amounts of fluids and take the medications as instructed. General rules are to take all hypertensive medication and platelet inhibitors (aspirin and clopidogrel) and avoid taking nonsteriodal medications (such as Ibuprofen) for twenty four hours prior to the procedure. Patients with diabetes who take insulin should cut their doses in half and hold their oral hypoglycemic medications the morning of the procedure. Metformin is an oral hypoglycemic agent of particular importance. You should not take metformin the morning of the procedure and it is recommended not to be restarted until it is clear no kidney failure occurred from the dye used in the procedure.

Warfarin is a very strong blood thinner that should be stopped at least three days prior to the catheterization (a doctor should guide the drug withdrawl).

Some patients with mechanical heart valves have to be hospitalized when stopping warfarin.

Patients should have someone accompany them going home and staying the night. Patients should bring their insurance cards, medications and write down questions they have concerning their procedure. Patients should inform the medical staff if they have any allergies to dye, kidney problems or thyroid problems. Due to the nature of the work, emergency procedures often create schedule delays and realizing they can occur often lessen the anxiety which can build up waiting for one's procedure.

Who are the Staff in the Cath Lab that I will be in contact with?

The catheterization lab has a multidisciplinary team of medical staff. Front office staff will check patients in a reception area to obtain demographic and insurance information. The team consists of invasive cardiologists, interventional cardiologists, cardiology fellows (doctors in training), nurse practitioners, physician assistants, registered nurses, nursing assistants, and cardiovascular technicians all of whom have specialized training.

What can I expect to happen in the Catheterization procedure?

The doctors (or their surrogates) and nurses will do a pre-procedure work up consisting of taking a medical history, performing a physical exam and reviewing blood tests, electrocardiograms and other non-invasive tests.

The staff will insert intravenous lines, place EKG leads, place oxygen monitors, place blood pressure monitors and possibly insert a urinary catheter. They will review the procedure with the patient including the risks and benefits and obtain an informed consent.

The patient may be given a mild oral or an intravenous sedative. The team in the procedure room monitors the patient's blood pressure, heart rate and rhythm, breathing, fluid intake and urine output. A local anesthetic is given into the skin at the site (the leg or the arm) of the initial tube insertion. The X-ray equipment and catheters are also being monitored. A log of the events occurring in the case is kept and the x-ray pictures of the arteries are recorded and stored.

The post-procedure care involves: monitoring the vital signs, checking the arterial entry site for bleeding, checking peripheral pulses, assessing urine output, assessing the post procedure electrocardiogram, assessing the level of consciousness and pain assessments. Depending on the size of the initial tube that was used and if a sealing device was able to be placed, bed rest will be needed from two to six hours. Rest and low level activity is generally recommended for the first three days after the procedure. A shower can be taken twenty four hours after the procedure; however a bath should be avoided for three days.

What are the Possible Complications that Can Occur in the Cath Lab?

Extensive analysis of complications in more than 200,000 patients indicates the following risks for a diagnostic catheterization: death <.2%, heart attack <.05%, stroke <.07%, serious heart rhythm problems < 0.5%, and major vascular complications (bleeding requiring transfusion or injury requiring surgery) < 1.0%.[3]

Cardiac catheterizations are currently performed safely in hospitals with and without cardiac surgery backup. In hospitals with cardiac surgery, essentially all patients can undergo invasive studies safely. Full support services include not only cardiac surgery but also vascular surgery, nephrology and dialysis, neurology, hematology, and specialized imaging. [4]

The American College of Cardiology has set forth volume guidelines in an attempt to confirm adequate skill and quality for both the laboratory and for the individual operators. Each adult diagnostic cardiac catheterization laboratory should perform at least 300 cases a year and adult interventional laboratories should ideally do at least 400 cases per year. [4,5] An invasive cardiologist should perform at least 150 diagnostic cases per year and interventional cardiologist should perform at least 75 interventional cases per year. [5] Outcomes related to complications for diagnostic catheterizations should be very low, less than one percent. Major complications (death, heart attack, stroke, and emergency surgery) from interventional procedures should be less than three percent. [4]

A good resource for patients undergoing a catheterization procedure is the American College of Cardiology web site at *www.cardiosmart.org*.

References:

1. Thom T, Hasse N, Rosamond W, et al. American Heart Association Statistics Committee and Stroke Statistics Subcommittee. American Heart Association statistical update: heart disease and stroke statistics-2006 update. January 1, 2006.
2. Brunwald E. Heart Disease A Textbook of Cardiovascular Medicine. 5[th]ed. Philadelphia, W.B. Saunders Company, 1997:4.
3. Kern, MJ. The Cardiac Catheterization Handbook. 3rd ed. Mosby, Inc., 1999:6-8
4. Bashore et al., ACC/SCA&I Clinical Expert Consensus Document on Catheterization Laboratory Standards JACC Vol. 37, NO. 8, June 2001:2170-214
5. Watson S, Gorski K. Invasive Cardiology A Manual for Cath Lab Personnel. 2nd ed. Royal Oak, Michigan, Physicians' Press, 2005:93

Chemical Dependency Services

Stanley Yancovitz, MD, Ed Salsitz, MD,
Kevin Maccoll, MA, Patti Juliana, MSW

We know that millions of Americans misuse or are dependent on alcohol or drugs. Most of them have families who suffer the consequences of living with this illness. We believe that drug and alcohol dependence disorders are medical conditions that can be effectively treated. The first step is to have the courage and honesty to admit to having an addiction problem. Sometimes, family members help the person find the motivation for treatment. Treatment programs will help you build on this first step, and give you the tools to overcome your addiction problems.

There are a full range of treatment services to help you recover from the disease of addiction. Most patients are first admitted to a detoxification unit for the treatment and prevention of withdrawal symptoms, resulting from stopping drug use. After the detoxification is completed, patients may be transferred to either an in-patient or out-patient rehabilitation units for ongoing care and recovery.

What can I expect when I am admitted to the drug detoxification program?

The word *detoxification* is a common expression in addiction treatment. A more accurate term is *withdrawal management*. Most of the drugs which patients are using when they seek "detox" are alcohol, heroin, Xanax, Vicodan and cocaine, for example. When patients stop using these drugs, they develop a withdrawal syndrome. Continued drug use is often an attempt to alleviate the symptoms of withdrawal. Withdrawal from some drugs, like heroin or prescription opioids, can be very painful and unpleasant. Withdrawal from alcohol or benzodiazepam can be dangerous. You have probably heard of "DTs", which is a symptom of severe alcohol withdrawal. The goals of detoxification are to provide safe and humane withdrawal from substances and to foster the patient's entry into long-term treatment and recovery.

When you are admitted you will have a comprehensive clinical assessment. You will be seen by the nursing and medical staff shortly after arriving on the unit. There will be many questions asked about your past and current medical concerns. This is done in order for the treatment team to make an accurate assessment of your medical needs. At this time the medical staff may determine that you need medications to safely withdraw from the drugs and/or alcohol you have been taking.

Although you may be tired when you are admitted, this initial evaluation is very important, so please be patient. We need to determine what treatment is needed to prevent withdrawal symptoms or other complications of withdrawal. Sometimes the initial assessment and treatment may have to be revised in the days you spend on the detoxification unit. You will be monitored frequently for any signs of withdrawal, but please report any symptoms to the nurse.

You will also be assigned a substance abuse counselor who will work with you to develop your treatment plan. This will be the course of action that you will follow during your hospitalization. It may include individual and group counseling, health lectures, medication management and attendance at self-help meetings. Psychiatric evaluation and support are also provided during your stay. You and your counselor will be developing your aftercare plans. These plans may include further treatment in a residential or outpatient program, which is a very important part of your treatment. The aftercare plans will help you in your recovery from substance abuse.

Although detoxification is sometimes a little uncomfortable, it is only the first step. Many patients have tried to "detox," many times on their own, and have had many admissions for "detox." Addiction is a chronic and relapsing disease. It can be successfully treated, but it often takes repeated episodes of treatment. Don't be discouraged—most patients go through a series of "detoxs" before they move on to a longer lasting recovery.

How can I assure my best outcome in the drug detoxification unit?

We encourage you to be proactive in your treatment. By following the treatment plan, attending the daily activities and meeting with the members of your treatment team, it will help ensure that your stay is a successful one. Remember, you have taken a courageous step in addressing your substance abuse problem and your journey toward recovery is a day at a time.

For a variety of reasons, patients sometimes "sign out" of the program before their treatment is completed. Addiction is a difficult disease, and staying in the hospital can be difficult, especially if you have a lot of problems—personal, family, legal and work problems. But, if you "stick" with a program of recovery, you can gradually put this disease into remission.

If you have problems on the "outside," the entire staff will try and help you solve your problems while you continue in treatment. Often, when patients "sign out," it increases the chance of relapse. So, please let us try to help, and stay until your treatment ends. That is the best way to assure your best outcome.

What medications will be used in the drug detoxification unit?

Medications are used to detoxify a person from the drugs or alcohol that they have been abusing. The medical team will determine which medication and how it will be administered to you. In general, people using opiates (e.g. Heroin, Oxycontin) will be given methadone or buprenorphine. If you are abusing alcohol the medication given may be Phenobarbital. Sometimes, no medication may be necessary when alcohol is stopped. For benzodiazepines (Valium, Xanax, Ativan), Phenobarbital or clonazepam are used. We carefully monitor patients for seizures during this withdrawal. For tobacco addiction, we offer nicotine patches and/or gum. Since smoking is prohibited throughout the detoxification program, we recommend the use of these alternatives.

A detoxification schedule will be written and you will be given tapering dosages of the prescribed medications. During this time the treatment team will closely monitor your reaction to the detoxification medications. It is imperative that you inform the treatment team immediately if you are feeling ill.

How do I know I am getting the best care?

There are two ways you can know this. The first is by asking what services are available after detoxification. Detoxification isn't substance abuse treatment but is one part of a continuum of care for substance-related disorders. The last step in the process of detoxification is helping the person get ready for and enter into ongoing treatment services. In order to do that, a program has to either provide the service or have good relationships with other treatment programs that provide other services such as the inpatient and outpatient services that are described below (Aftercare). It is important to also have good linkages with therapeutic communities, where people can stay for long-term care, and supportive housing organizations.

The other way you can know if you are getting the best care is to look for licensing and. For example, our programs are licensed by the **New York State Office of Alcohol and Substance Abuse Services** as well as **The Joint Commission.** These two organizations provide oversight and ensure that the best possible care is being provided by our medical center. All our staff including physicians, physician's assistants, nurses and counselors are licensed and /or credentialed by their respective professional organizations.

What should I do if I have concerns about my care?

You will be assigned a nurse and a counselor upon admission. Ask to see either one with your concerns. If they are not available please ask any staff member for assistance. Each detoxification unit has a nurse manager and a social work supervisor assigned to the unit. Please see them if your concerns are not resolved.

Aftercare

What happens after detoxification is most important. Plans for aftercare were mentioned in the paragraph about treatment plans. Our program offers two options for continuing care for people who have completed detoxification: inpatient and outpatient rehabilitation.

Inpatient rehabilitation is the best next step in treatment. The inpatient rehabilitation unit has many group meetings, individual counseling, mutual help meetings, spirituality, and family treatment services. This is an active program, and you will be busy with the work of recovery for most of the day. Your on-going medical needs will be coordinated by the physician's assistant, along with the nursing staff. You will receive health education information to keep you safer and healthier when you are discharged. Again, plans will be made for longer term and ongoing care after your discharge. Please remember that addiction is treatable, but not curable. Continuing care, such as attending the outpatient rehabilitation service is very important.

Head and Neck Surgery

Mark Persky, M.D.

If I need surgery, when do I need to be admitted to the hospital or get outpatient surgery?

Head and neck surgery has evolved over the past several years. Minimally invasive procedures have been introduced for some surgical approaches and this often results in faster recovery as well as the possibility of performing your procedure as an outpatient. The ultimate decision concerning the surgical procedure or need for hospitalization is made after a thorough discussion between the patient and physician. Most importantly, each case must be individually considered with evaluation of the medical co-morbidities, possibility of postoperative swelling and/or pain causing difficulty in breathing/swallowing, necessity for surgical drains, and availability of necessary assistance at home.

Procedures involving major tumor resections, extensive reconstruction, or considerable airway manipulation will most often require postoperative inpatient care and observation. Sometimes, a temporary tracheostomy will be necessary for safe airway control or a feeding tube will be inserted through the nose and into the stomach to provide adequate postoperative nutrition. This will require an inpatient hospitalization. Although there is more pressure on surgeons by insurance companies to perform surgeries as outpatient procedures, individual medical considerations may warrant that a physician contact the insurance company to obtain a medical review and thereby obtain permission for inpatient surgery.

What can I expect about my hospitalization?

The patient should expect the hospital to be clean, efficient, and provide the necessary staff and technology to provide a comfortable, caring and professional level of medical and postoperative care. Patients are required to check into the hospital, usually on the day of surgery, and the process prior to surgery should be as comforting as possible, especially considering the anxiety the patient and their families are experiencing. After the demographic and insurance data are confirmed, a nurse will interview the patient and review their medical history as well as make sure that the patient understands the proposed surgical procedure. The surgeon and the anesthesiologist will also meet the patient to answer any last minute questions or to clarify outstanding issues. The anesthesiologist will describe the procedures to be followed as the patient is brought into the operating room, receives an intravenous line and has monitoring equipment applied. The patient will also know when the intravenous anesthetic agent will be administered. Upon awakening from the anesthesia, the patient will be brought to the recovery room where skilled nurses will monitor the patient's progress. Occasionally, patients experience nausea and pain related to the anesthesia drugs and surgery. This can be managed with a variety of effective medications. When a patient is transferred to their hospital room, the nursing staff will be fully advised of the patient's status, which should result in specific protocols of care tailored to the patient's needs. Effective control of pain is crucial and the patient's activity and dietary needs are monitored. Intravenous lines and possible urinary catheters, if present, will be attended to. With head and neck procedures, airway observation is of special importance. The staff should be responsive to the patient's needs. Patients with tracheostomies will often not be able to verbally communicate, therefore the availability of writing instruments is important. Any perceived problems with your care should be discussed with your attending physician or the nurse responsible for your care.

Who will be the members of my health care team in the hospital?

There are many teams involved with your hospital care and their interaction is important in providing you with safe, comfortable and efficient care during your hospitalization. If you are in a medical center involved with physician education and training, there may be resident physicians of various levels of seniority who are closely involved with your care. These are hard working young doctors who are a constant presence in the hospital and will communicate with your physician about your ongoing hospital care. In many hospitals, nurse practitioners and physician assistants will also be involved in the care that your doctor has outlined. The nursing team will consist of registered nurses, licensed practical nurses, and nurses aides who are constantly surveying your progress and needs-administering medications, taking care of drains and wounds including tracheostomies and feeding tubes, monitoring vital signs such as temperature, blood pressure, pulse, respiration rate, coordinating the various services involved in your care, and providing for your personal hygiene. To provide for your needs there are a myriad of other personnel: social workers, technicians, therapists and administrators. Unfortunately, in the busy and complicated world of the hospital, there may be lapses in the coordination of all of these services and activities. If you perceive any problem, please discuss this with your doctor or nurse.

Will my doctor see me every day?

Your doctor should see you each day of your hospitalization. Often, doctors have colleagues who participate in the care of each other's hospitalized patients. All of these physicians will be aware of your medical and surgical situation and will be able to provide the necessary treatment. Prior to any hospital care, your doctor should discuss your case with other physicians who may participate in your care or if there may be an unavoidable absence due to professional or academic activities or vacations.

Many of the larger medical centers have training programs for resident physicians who are studying to become experts in specific fields of medicine or surgery. They represent an important aspect of your care. A member of the resident team staffs the hospital 24 hours a day and they will also be visiting you to evaluate your status and define any needs. They represent an important extension and compliment to your physician's care.

Who will be doing my surgery?

Your physician will be performing your surgery but there are many procedures that require assistance. These assistants may be the resident physicians who will be closely supervised by your surgeon during the surgery. Often there may be procedures requiring more than one assistant. Occasionally, there may be a nurse practitioner or a physician's assistant who has the necessary skills to assist the surgeon. If you have any concerns about who participates in your surgery or their roles during the operation, fee free to ask. There will also be others in the operating room—anesthesiologists, nurses and technicians—who provide important skills for your operative care.

What should I do if I have a question or concern about my care?

Any questions or concerns should be immediately brought to the attention of the doctors or nurses participating in your care. The focus of all hospital personnel should be patient care. If you encounter any difficulties or perceive any danger or compromise in your care, this issue should be brought to the attention of either your physician or nursing team. Sometimes, there are unanticipated complications or problems that occur and this should be thoroughly discussed with you and your family. If there is a particular problem with your care that you feel has not been adequately addressed, the hospital will provide a patient care representative to advocate on your behalf. A thorough preoperative discussion of hospital care considerations and possible complications related to your surgery should anticipate most aspects of your experience during your hospital stay.

How do I know when I am ready to go home?

If you required hospital admission for your surgery, your anticipated hospital stay and recuperation should have been one of the points of discussion between you and your surgeon. The site and extent of your surgical procedure will impact the length of your hospitalization. Before a patient is discharged, it is important that there is control of postoperative pain and discomfort, adequate recovery of nutritional intake and resolution of any breathing difficulties and recovery of ambulation and self-care. If a prolonged presence of a tracheostomy or feeding tube is necessary, the expert nursing care should educate you on managing these issues. Occasionally, the patient may be discharged with the necessary assistance of concerned family members and/or visiting nurse services. Sometimes, discharge to a skilled nursing facility is part of the postoperative recuperation. The timing of the hospital discharge and the need for any instructions or postoperative care arrangements, including any necessary home care equipment, should be discussed with the patient and family as the patient's progress is monitored. Last-minute discharge notification is unwarranted since the patient needs the necessary emotional preparation for hospital discharge. Any involved family members should be included in this discussion.

Integrative Medicine

Woodson Merrell, MD

Why Do I Hear So Much About Integrative Medicine?

Going into the hospital is always a stressful time, both for patients and their families. There are a number of ways that the stress can be managed. Many of these can also improve the medical outcomes at the same time. The focus needs to be not on treating the diagnosis, but on the whole patient: not on reducing a set of symptoms, but on promoting the healing process that will lead to a stronger person after the procedure. The crux of this is good communication between the doctor and the patient. But you will be a step ahead if you choose a hospital that focuses on providing supportive healing services in addition to standard medical care.

Twenty years ago there was scant evidence to support many innovative services, but over the last 10-12 years there has been an explosion of quality information to guide providers and their patients as to how to maximize not only hospital outcomes—but patients' health in general. While of course this approach should be standard of practice for all medical care, it has not been a priority since the age of specialization came in the 1960s. Cutbacks in insurance reimbursements and governmental funding combined with ever-escalating costs have lead to reduction in staff and services in many hospitals, put further stress on the existing staff, and reduced the time spent between staff and patients. Time pressures have become huge. A study in 1999 showed that the average time to interruption by a doctor in an initial patient interview was 23 seconds, and the majority of patients never got to detail the reason they came in for treatment. (1) The current era of integrative medicine seeks to help rebalance this inequity

As stated by former Chancellor of Duke University, Ralph Snyderman, MD and Director of the University of Arizona's Program in Integrative Medicine, Andrew Weil, MD "The chassis is broken, and the wheels are coming off . . . . integrative medicine should be a cornerstone of the urgently needed reconfiguration of our increasingly dysfunctional system of health care." (2)

Now over 30% of US and Canadian medical school deans have pledged that the integrative medicine approach will be the standard at their medical school and residency training programs through membership in the national Consortium of Academic Health Centers for Integrative Medicine (CAHCIM). Its "mission is to help transform healthcare through rigorous scientific studies, new models of clinical care, and innovative educational programs that integrate biomedicine, the complexity of human beings, the intrinsic nature of healing and the rich diversity of therapeutic systems." (3) As the paper by Snyderman and Weil states, "the success of the (integrative medicine) movement will be signaled by dropping the adjective" (2).

What exactly is integrative medicine?

A lot of confusion has ensued the last few decades as holistic medicine morphed into alternative medicine, then to complementary medicine and finally to integrative medicine. According to CAHCIM, the definition of integrative medicine is "the practice of medicine that reaffirms the importance of relationship between practitioner and patient, focuses on the whole person, is informed by evidence, and makes use of all appropriate therapeutic approaches to achieve optimal health and healing." (3)

The key concept here is that Integrative medicine is NOT alternative medicine. Alternative medicine implies that the remedy used is done so instead of conventional medicine. Another term that is utilized for this new era in healthcare is complementary. This denotes therapies that can be used in conjunction with conventional, that complement each other. This is a useful term, but today most providers prefer to use the term integrative. This describes the optimum approach—one that considers all therapeutic options both conventional, alternative and complementary and chooses the one or ones that will work best with fewest side effects. This is regardless of which tradition they come from: complementary/alternative, indigenous (including Traditional Chinese or Ayurvedic medicine going back 1000s of years), and conventional.

What are the Principles of Integrative Medicine?

Integrative medicine seeks to help reconfigure health care through four principles:

1) Relationship-centered: not doctor or even patient-centric: being focused on the relationship between patient and care-giver—as a partnership.

2) Empowering the patient: helping develop the tools for each patient to take charge as much as possible for their own healing progress

3) Optimal Wellness: having this as the goal and not disease or symptom alleviation or cessation—having a total person focus: mind-body and spirit as the goal

4) Conventional Framework: using the foundation of conventional western bioscientific medicine, with complementary/alternative and indigenous approaches blended in whenever appropriate

What Are the Fundamentals of the Integrative Medicine Approach?

First and foremost, integrative medicine seeks to maximize each person's life-style, through emphasis on:

- stress management
- exercise
- social connectivity
- proper rest
- diet/nutritional status

When life-style changes alone are insufficient, therapeutic approaches and modalities that have been shown to be helpful to effect progress toward optimal health include:

- mind-body practices/stress reduction
- nutrition (diet) and nutritional supplements
- herbs (botanicals)
- body work (i.e. massage, chiropractic)
- acupuncture
- indigenous healing systems
- energy medicine (reiki, therapeutic touch, qi gong; also homeopathy)
- spirituality (prayer, connectivity)
- healing arts (ie music, dance, art therapies)
- nature (i.e. plant and pet therapies)
- movement therapy (i.e. tai chi, yoga)

Is Integrative Medicine Safe and Efficacious?

All therapies need to be as safe as possible. Certainly the more invasive the procedure and the worse the underlying condition, the greater there is for potential adverse consequences. Knowledge of the relative risks and benefits of any procedure needs to be clear between provider and patient. No therapy can ultimately be guaranteed to be completely safe. Somewhere someone is sensitive to most every intervention: thousands of people die every year from aspirin's side-effects, yet it is certainly not going to be taken off the market (nor should it be): it just needs to be used carefully and appropriately. Integrative medicine has the same standards as all medical care: use the safest remedy possible.

Every therapy should be the most effective one available. But again, as the risks go up, with a more effective therapy, the balance needs to be carefully weighed.

Integrative medicine is subject to the exact same standards. Over 20 states in the United States have Alternative (sic) Medicine Practice Acts. These state that a practitioner can enter into a relationship with each patient utilizing any therapeutic intervention based only on whether the therapy is the 1) safest, 2) most effective, 3) if unconventional, informed consent needs to be given, and 4) if unconventional, nothing in conventional medicine is better. Whether the therapy is one of those listed above (coming from complementary or indigenous traditions), antibiotics, steroids or surgery, the only standard for practice should be what is best (safest and most effective) for each individual patient.

The bar for safety certainly goes higher when a patient enters a hospital. The drugs are usually stronger, the patient often weaker, and procedures and surgical interventions carry added risks. Patients MUST tell their providers, and providers MUST be taught to ask, what each and every patient is taking—ideally at least two weeks before being admitted.

Should I Consider the Use of Supplements (Nutritional or Herbal) (4,5,6)?

In general, all non-prescription supplements must be stopped at least one week before admission—unless specifically cleared for use by one's admitting doctor.

There are many supplements available now that can positively impact health. Many of them work by having anti-oxidant or anti-inflammatory effects on the body—helping it heal, and protecting it from future damage. But the reason these substances work is that they have active biological properties: the chemicals contained within them have an impact on the body's functioning. While in many cases the benefits of these supplements have been worked out, the potential risks may not yet be fully realized—especially in a precarious medical condition. This is especially important in considering potential interactions with anesthesia and medications. Some herbs are known to interfere with the body's ability to metabolize drugs (such as St. John's Wort, and even grapefruit juice!): more will be identified in the years ahead. And a number of supplements are known to increase bleeding tendencies; especially fish and flax oil, vitamin E and ginkgo biloba. Unlike some critical medications (for diabetes, hypertension, antibiotics, etc.) there is virtually no non-prescription supplement that cannot safely be stopped temporarily. Always ask: don't take them without your doctor's explicit OK.

Can I Use Integrative Therapies While I am in the Hospital?

While some integrative techniques and therapies may be inappropriate for use in the hospital, there are many that have an evidence basis to consider incorporating in conventional hospital care. Some of these have been shown to be safe and can improve patient quality of life and outcomes. These include:

1) *Mind-body techniques:* This represents a family of therapeutic modalities that while similar, have different approaches to invoking each person's innate healing abilities (7)

   - Meditation (8,9,10)
     Meditation involves sitting quietly and focusing on one thought that will let all others float away. The thought can be a sound or mantra such as the soothing sound Om or any sound that is pleasant; a word such as peace or calm; an image, such as surf on the beach or walking through a forest with the sunlight breaking through the trees, or your own breath. The thought you focus on is less relevant than using this device to allow your conscious thoughts to drift away—and leave you in a peaceful state, with your mind quieted. There are dozens of studies attesting to the power of meditation to not only promote relaxation, but promote healing—especially an improvement in the nervous and immune systems.

   - Self-hypnosis (11, 12)
     I am referring to self-hypnosis here, to differentiate it from the more commonly known stage hypnosis. Clinical hypnosis endeavors to help you change thought and behavior patterns. It is commonly used, usually by psychotherapists to help with eating, smoking, and phobias. But it is equally useful and used to help with pain and functional problems—shortness of breath, headaches and insomnia. For patients facing hospitalization, especially where pain may be anticipated it should be considered for use. It has been shown to be especially helpful in children for reducing anxiety and pain.

- Imagery (13, 14, 15)

  Imagery is akin to meditation. However with imagery, as opposed to using a thought or image to allow the mind to clear, with imagery, one develops a specific image to promote healing with a specific problem. An example would be to imagine that a white light is suffusing a problem spot (ulcer, cancer, pain site, etc), providing healing energy to help take away not only the symptoms from the condition but the condition itself. The images can be quite elaborate, entailing a process ending up in the organ, or can be simpler, just focusing in on the problem area and using images of a well-body to promote healing. One of my favorite studies had burn patients imagining they were in a freezing place in the Arctic, as their bandages are being changed: the technique was shown to dramatically reduce the pain of the procedure.

- Biofeedback (16,17)

  Biofeedback is what I call meditation for engineers. It invokes the same relaxation response as with imagery and meditation, but allows the practitioner to receive biological feedback (bio-feedback—usually through earphones with a tone) as to how they are progressing with their attempt to relax. This usually involves having a monitor placed on two fingertips or the forehead, which measures the difference in electrical resistance between the two points. This difference has been shown to correlate with the brain' alpha, or calming waves. The lower the resistance—the less stressed is the brain and nervous system, and the lower the tone heard through the headset. This allows one to monitor the relaxation results. Studies have shown biofeedback to be especially useful in stress and pain management, headache (including migraine) asthma, insomnia, and pain

- Breathwork/Yoga (16)

  Simply focusing on relaxing breaths can make a huge difference. Especially when stressed, we tend to hold our breath, or at the least breathe very shallow. Try it right now: sit comfortably, let the air flow in smoothly, (preferably using the diaphragm for abdominal breathing rather than the overworked chest muscles). Breathe in to a count of 4, hold the breath for a count of one, breathe out to a count of four, pause again for a count, then repeat. Doing this even four times will allow you to noticeably feel more relaxed—and let the overworked sympathetic nervous system have a chance to slow down. Do this every hour if you can.

2) *Acupuncture* (18,19,20,21)

Acupuncture has been in use continuously for 2,000 years, with its practices having been codified in a formal training manual 1,800 years ago. Research over the last 30 years has attested to its ability to alter many of the body's systems: neurotransmitters (including serotonin and dopamine, positively affecting mood), stress hormones (adrenaline and cortisone), pain perception (through raising endorphin and blocking substance P levels), muscle spasm (by inhibiting the reflex arc that goes from the muscle to the spine then back out producing spasm), and inflammation (improving the balance of cells and chemicals that reduce rather than increase inflammatory processes such as arthritis). Acupuncture is done by inserting a sterilized (one-time use) needle through the skin into specific acupuncture points. These lie along nervous system meridians that were worked out over hundreds of years, and practiced with little change for literally millennia. The patient barely feels anything from the needles—they are very thin with a sharp tip that penetrates the skin usually painlessly. Occasionally when the needle finds a particularly tense point a mild aching sensation is felt—known in Traditional Chinese Medicine as de-Qi. (pronounced de chee). Acupuncture sessions last 15-30 minutes. Since points are present throughout the body (over 400—originally 365), if a patient has particular areas that cannot be accessed or touched, distant points can be used. Acupuncture's best use in the hospital is for pain and stress control, but any of the problems described above can be addressed, as well as functional problems such as irritable bowel, sinus and chest congestion, and headaches. Acupuncture can be administered by either physicians or licensed acupuncturists (L.Ac. or OMD {Oriental Medical Doctors}).

3) *Body work*

i. Massage and Physical Therapy (22,23,24,25,26)

Physical therapists use many massage techniques as well as other therapies (deep heat, ultrasound, manipulation, exercise training) under the direction of a physician. Their work in the hospital often focuses on people with serious neuromuscular and musculoskeletal problems: most commonly coming from strokes, accidents, and neurodegenerative diseases. Massage therapists are well-trained to do work with musculoskeletal problems—and in most states also have a license to do so, but with a more limited scope of practice than a physical therapist. Their work focuses on working out tension within the muscular structures, which usually also provides relief from stress. There are a number of different massage techniques, including Swedish (more relaxing, stroking massage), shiatsu (harder into tender trigger points), and sports (deeper kneading of muscles and tendons). Another kind of body therapy that is offered in some hospitals is Reflexology. This is particularly safe for most patients—as it involves work only with the foot.

- Chiropractic/Osteopathy (27,28,29)
  Most hospitals will not offer these therapies, as they involve active manipulation of the patient's spine and adjacent tissues. Osteopaths (D.O.) and chiropractors (D.C.) are both doctors: unlike physical therapists and massage therapists, they can diagnose and treat any patient on their own. Hospitals that do credential them for inpatient work often limit their scope of practice, as spinal manipulation for physically challenged patients has heightened risks that make it sometime best to use these techniques when the situation is not as critical, usually in the outpatient setting. Physical therapists can do work close to these in the interim but especially for patients who have had the work done before, and by providers trained to work with more difficult hospitalized patients, there is definitely a role for this approach in hospitals, particularly with musculoskeletal problems.

4) *Healing Touch/Energy Medicine*

- Reiki, Therapeutic touch, Qi gong, Healing touch (30,31)
  Though their adherents certainly view these practices differently, they are sufficiently similar that I will review them as a group. The word touch is actually a misnomer. These are practices that involve transmitting energy from one individual to another, usually without touch. We all radiate energy—in the case of the heart, detectable up to 12 feet away. A simple way to understand the use of energy transmission in healing touch is to place your palm about an inch away from another person and see if you can feel heat emanating from them. The same can be done in reverse, with your palm's energy being felt by the other person. While these practices seem ephemeral, there are studies (particularly in T.T. and reiki) attesting to benefits from these practices—especially in promoting relaxation. They are often performed by nurses.

- Homeopathy (32)

  Homeopathy is still a controversial practice. While it is FDA-approved (grandfathered in when the FDA was first formed) and is based on double-blind research to determine its remedies, the fact that the homeopathic substances work when they are diluted past Avogadro's number (the dilution beyond which there should be nothing left of the original material substance) makes its use difficult to accept, much less recommend by many physicians. At its most fundamental level, homeopathy has to be considered as energy medicine. Placing the ultra-diluted sugar pellets under the tongue effects a change in the body—explained by homeopaths to a vaccine-like mechanism of introducing a small amount of a substance to stimulate the body to react against that very substance's effects if given in full potency. In my review paper on the subject, I point out that while the mechanisms of action still remain to be elucidated, the proof is in the pudding—are there studies that show that it works? And the answer to this is a qualified yes. Qualified as there are as many negative as positive studies in the mainstream literature. For the same reason that critics do not believe in homeopathy—because there is nothing there, it is nearly impossible for it to cause harm. Indeed, these sublingual, sugar pellets can be taken before and after surgery, In New York City, many plastic surgeons' pre-operative instructions recommend homeopathic arnica to help reduce bruising and swelling.

5) *Art therapies*: music, art, dance, writing (journaling) (33,34,35)

   The last decade has seen a wonderful increase in arts therapies offered within hospitals. Many hospitals have formal departments. (Beth Israel Medical Center's (BIMC) Louis Armstrong Department of Music Therapy is one of the top programs in the nation).While music therapy sometimes means someone coming to the room or in a group gathering to provide live music, most often music therapy entails listening to music on CDs that have been specifically made to enhance healing for patients going through difficult times. Dance therapy is often done for more mobile outpatients. Art therapy and journaling provide (especially the more infirmed) patients the opportunity to let out their stresses through an artistic or expository vehicle that can be very liberating and healing. You don't need a formal therapist to do this—try yourself to write out your thoughts and feelings, and to listen to music that transports you to a beautiful, peaceful place. Art therapies have specific, usually hospital-based training programs.

6) *Movement therapy*: tai chi, yoga (36,37,38,39, 40, 41)

Yoga and tai chi have been around for thousands of years. They have become increasingly available to the medical community. They both involve specific bodily positions and careful movements while focusing on the breath. Indeed, breathwork is at the core of bringing up one's energy—described in yoga as prana and tai chi as Qi. Yoga in particular can be done seated, or even lying down, with very simple exercises. For the bed-bound, yoga may even mean just working with the breath, with as good posture as possible. Tai chi is used more when one can stand and move about. Tai chi has been shown to help with imbalance, and yoga with impaired breathing, and both have been shown to improve immune system functioning. Most teachers of these disciplines are certified by training institutes but do not necessarily have a formal medical license.

7) Nature

i.   Pet therapy. (42)

Increasingly, hospitals have trained dogs to serve as companions for hospitalized patients, including in the Intensive Care Units. It is wonderful to see the smile come over patients going through grueling medical procedures when a pet comes in to share their time. Ask if this is available to you—usually through the Volunteer Department.

•   Plant therapy (43)

Hospitals are increasingly recognizing the power that comes from connecting with nature while in stressful(and often drab) institutional environments. Of course bringing flowers to patients has been a sign of support and love for centuries. But making the commitment to have plants available to patients from the institution is a welcome change, and another aid to reducing stress and providing connection with our inner healing resources.

8) *Aromatherapy* (44,45,46,47,48)

This is the use of essential oils—plant extracts distilled down to the oil essence within the plant. These essences not only smell wonderful, but have been shown in studies to have specific heath properties. In the hospital they are mainly used for their ability to reduce stress and tension. They can be applied (diluted) as a massage oil, or put in a room diffuser. One technique (the "M-technique" taught by Jane Buckle, RN) uses the oils in a specific hand massage that is especially useful for patients who cannot be moved or even touched in most of their body. Lavender is probably the most popular and best studied of the oils, though others such as clary sage and peppermint are also popular.

9) *Spirituality* (49,50,51,52,53)

Connecting with one's spiritual roots while going through difficult times provides immense solace, and has been shown to increases our ability to heal. There are hundreds of studies on religion, prayer and spirituality by such luminaries in the field as Drs. Harold Koenig, Jeffrey Levin and Larry Dossey. While atheists can certainly utilize many of the practices listed above—including mind-body ones, there is no doubt that feeling connected to a higher power not only makes us feel more comforted, but puts in motion emotional and physical processes within us that enhance healing. There is increasing emphasis on insuring that patients receive support for their own spiritual resources. Most hospitals have had chaplains for decades. There have been a number of peer-reviewed studies showing the improvement in recovery, notably in AIDS and CCU patients, even when people were prayed for anonymously (unknown even to the patients). BIMC even has a special Zen Buddhist chaplaincy program, incorporating the spiritual practices of this philosophy with many other religious traditions. I like the statement by Larry Dossey that knowing what we do now about prayer and spirituality, not to recommend prayer in the 21st century should be considered malpractice.

Integrative medicine is the future of medicine. And it is here now. The key is to have a provider who is knowledgeable about the therapy being considered. Many modalities are available through in-hospital, credentialed practitioners. Some therapies even have full hospital departments (music, art). Increasingly pharmacists are trained to know what supplements may be safe. Ask before you go. Press for care that is integrative—or at least care in a facility that supports integrative services. (54)

Footnotes and Bibliography

(1)   *Marvel MK, Epstein RM,* Flowers K, Beckiman HB, Soliciting the patient's agenda: have we improved?, *JAMA 1999 Jan 20;281(3):283-7.*

(2)   *Snyderman Ralph & Weil Andrew, Integrative Medicine: Bringing Medicine Back to its Roots,* Arch Intern Med, Feb 25, 2002; 162(4): 395-97

(3)   *www.imconsortium.org*

(4)   *Javed F, et al.* Potential effects of herbal medicines and nutritional supplements on coagulation in ENT practice. *J Laryngol Otol. 2008 Feb;122(2):116-9.*

(5)   *Abebe W, Herbal medication: potential for adverse interactions with analgesic drugs, J Clin Pharm Ther.* 2002 Dec;27(6):391-401

(6)   *Ang-Lee MK, Moss J, Yuan CS, Herbal medicines and perioperative care JAMA.* 2001 Jul 11;286(2):208-16.

(7)   Marilyn Schlitz and Tina Amorok, *Consciousness and Healing*, Churchill Livingstone/Elsevier, 2005

(8)   Kabat-Zinn, Jonathan, *Wherever You Go There You Are: Mindfulness Meditation in Everyday Life*, Hyperion, 2003

(9)   *Pagnoni G, Cekic M, Age effects on gray matter volume and attentional performance in Zen meditation Neurobiol Aging*, 2007 Oct; 28(10): 1623-7.

(10)   *Kabat-Zinn J, Wheeler E, et al*, Influence of a mindfulness meditation-based stress reduction intervention on rates of skin clearing in patients with moderate to severe psoriasis undergoing phototherapy (UVB) and photochemotherapy (PUVA), *Psychosom Med 1998 Sep-Oct; 60(5): 625-32.*

(11)   *Wood C, Bioy A, Hypnosis and pain in children, J Pain Symptom Manage.* 2008 Apr; 35(4):437-46.

(12)   *Zeltzer L, LeBaron S,* Hypnosis and nonhypnotic techniques for reduction of pain and anxiety during painful procedures in children and adolescents with cancer, *J Pediatr. 1982 Dec; 101(6): 1032-5.*

(13)   Naparstek Belleruth, *Staying Well With Guided Imagery, Warner Books, 1994*

(14)   Naparstek Belleruth, *Health Journeys: Meditations to Relieve Stress*, (CD)

(15)   *Hoffman, H.G., Richards, T.L., et al, Using FMRI to study the neural correlates of virtual reality analgesia. CNS Spectrums*, 2006, *11*(1), 45-51. *[Available online: http://www.cnsspectrums.com/aspx/articledetail. aspx?articleid=449]*

(16)   Fried Robert, *Breath Well, Be Well: A Program to Relieve Stress, Anxiety, Asthma, Hypertension, Migraine and Other Disorders for Better Health*, John Wiley, 1999

(17)   *Reiner R.* Integrating a portable biofeedback device into clinical practice for patients with anxiety disorders: results of a pilot study, *Appl Psychophysiol Biofeedback 2008 Mar; 33(1): 55-61.*

(18)   Stux G, and Hammerschlag R, *Clinical Acupuncture: Scientific Basis*, Springer-Verlag, 2001

(19)   Han JS, *The Neurochemical Basis of Pain Relief by Acupuncture*, 1987

(20)   *Wonderling D, Vickers AJ, Grieve R, McCarney R, Cost effectiveness analysis of a randomised trial of acupuncture for chronic headache in primary care, BMJ.* 2004 Mar 27;328(7442):747.

(21)   *Vickers AJ, Rees RW, et al,* Acupuncture of chronic headache disorders in primary care: randomised controlled trial and economic analysis, *Health Technol Assess. 2004 Nov; 8(48):iii, 1-35.*

(22)   *Stringer J, Swindell R, Dennis M,* Massage in patients undergoing intensive chemotherapy reduces serum cortisol and prolactin, *Psychooncology 2008 Feb 26*

(23)   *Kaye AD, Kaye AJ, et al,* The effect of deep-tissue massage therapy on blood pressure and heart rate, *J Altern Complement Med. 2008 Mar;14(2):125-8.*

(24) *Mitchinson AR, Kim HM*, et al, Acute postoperative pain management using massage as an adjuvant therapy: a randomized trial, *Arch Surg.* 2007 Dec;142(12):1158-67

(25) *Chen LL, Su YC, Su CH, Lin HC, Kuo HW. Acupressure and meridian massage: combined effects on increasing body weight in premature infants. J Clin Nurs.* 2008 May;17(9):1174-81.

(26) *Quinn F, Hughes CM, Baxter GD, Reflexology in the management of low back pain: a pilot randomised controlled trial, Complement Ther Med.* 2008 Feb;16(1):3-8.

(27) *Bronfort G, Haas M, Evans RL, Bouter LM, Efficacy of spinal manipulation and mobilization for low back pain and neck pain: a systematic review and best evidence synthesis Spine J,* 2004 May-Jun;4(3):335-56.

(28) *Wilkey A, Gregory M, Byfield D, McCarthy PW.A comparison between chiropractic management and pain clinic management for chronic low-back pain in a national health service outpatient clinic J Altern Complement Med.* 2008 Jun;14(5):465-73.

(29) *Hurwitz EL,* et al, A randomized trial of chiropractic and medical care for patients with low back pain: eighteen-month follow-up outcomes from the UCLA low back pain study, *Spine. 2006 Mar 15;31(6):611-21*

(30) *Gronowicz GA,* et al, *Therapeutic touch stimulates the proliferation of human cells in culture, J Altern Complement Med.* 2008 Apr;14(3):233-9

(31) *MacKay N et al,* Autonomic nervous system changes during Reiki treatment: a preliminary study, *J Altern Complement Med. 2004 Dec; 10(6): 1077-81.*

(32) *Merrell, WC and Shalts, E, Homeopathy, Med Clin North Am,* Jan 2002, Jan; 86 (1): 47-62

(33) *Krout RE, The effects of single-session music therapy interventions on the observed and self-reported levels of pain control, physical comfort, and relaxation of hospice patients, Am J Hosp Pall Care,* 2001 Nov-Dec;18(6):383-90

(34) *Klassen JA, Liang Y, et al,* Music for pain and anxiety in children undergoing medical procedures: a systematic review of randomized controlled trials, *Ambul Pediatr. 2008 Mar-Apr;8(2):117-28.*

(35) *Smyth JM,* et al, *Expressive writing and post-traumatic stress disorder: effects on trauma symptoms, mood states, and cortisol reactivity. Br J Health Psychol.* 2008 Feb;13(Pt 1):85-93

(36) Yee Rodney, *Moving Toward Balance,* Rodale Press, 2004.

(37) *Pullen PR,* et al, *Effects of yoga on inflammation and exercise capacity in patients with chronic heart failure. J Card Fail,* 2008 Jun;14(5):407-13

(38) *DiStasio SA. Integrating yoga into cancer care, Clin J Oncol Nurs.* 2008 Feb;12(1):125-30

(39) *Danhauer SC,* et al, *Restorative yoga for women with ovarian or breast cancer: findings from a pilot study, J Soc Integr Oncol.* 2008 Spring; 6(2):47-58.

(40) *Li F, Harmer P,* et al, *Translation of an effective tai chi intervention into a community-based falls-prevention program, Am J Public Health.* 2008 Jul; 98(7):1195-8.

(41) *Wang JH,* Effects of tai chi exercise on patients with type 2 diabetes, *Med Sport Sci. 2008; 52: 230-8.*

(42) *Stasi MF, Amati D, et al,* Pet-therapy: a trial for institutionalized frail elderly patients, *Arch Gerontol Geriatr Suppl. 2004;(9):407-12*

(43) *Langer EJ, Rodin J,* The effects of choice and enhanced personal responsibility for the aged: a field experiment in an institutional setting, *J Pers Soc Psychol. 1976 Aug;34(2):191-8. (showing healing power of giving nursing home patients a plant)*

(42) *Fellowes D, Barnes K, Wilkinson S. Aromatherapy and massage for symptom relief in patients with cancer, Cochrane Database Syst Rev.* 2004;(2): CD002287

(45) *Moss M,* et al, *Aromas of rosemary and lavender essential oils differentially affect cognition and mood in healthy adults, Int J Neurosci.* 2003 Jan;113(1):15-38.

(46) *Moss M,* et al, *Modulation of cognitive performance and mood by aromas of peppermint and ylang-ylang, Int J Neurosci.* 2008 Jan;118(1):59-77

(47) *Pemberton E, Turpin PG, The effect of essential oils on work-related stress in intensive care unit nurses, Holist Nurs Pract.* 2008 Mar-Apr;22(2):97-102.

(48) Buckle, Jane, *Clinical Aromatherapy: Essential Oils in Practice,* Churchill Livingston, 2003

(49) Koenig, HC and Cohen, HJ, *The Link Between Religion and Health: Psychoneuroimunology and the Faith Factor,* Simon and Schuster, 2002

(50) Levin Jeffrey S, *God, Faith and Health: Exploring the Spirituality-Healing Connection,* John Wiley & Sons, 2001

(51) Dossey Larry, *Healing Words: The Power of Prayer and the Practice of Medicine,* Harper Collins, 1994

(52) *The Energy of Prayer,* Thich Nhat Hanh, Parallax Press, 2006

(53) *Mueller PS, et al, Religious involvement, spirituality, and medicine: implications for clinical practice, Mayo Clinic Proceedings,* 2001; 76: 1225-35. ("A prospective study of 232 people (age >55 years) undergoing elective heart surgery found that lack of participation in social groups and lack of strength or comfort from religion were the most consistent predictors of death, adjusted for age, previous cardiac surgery, and preoperative functional status.")

(54) Website for Beth Israel Medical Center's Continuum Center for Health and Healing: 800+ page compendium of information on integrative medical care: *www.healthandhealingny.org*

Kidney Disease

James Winchester, M.D.

What are my options and how can my safety be preserved?

You have just been told that you have kidney disease. The doctor was very informative but you still have a lot of questions, particularly about treatment and whether the condition is permanent or not.

Well, there are many kinds of kidney disease but usually the condition is divided into whether the disease arose suddenly (acute kidney injury) or more slowly (chronic kidney injury).

What is acute kidney injury?

Acute kidney injury is caused by many conditions ranging from dehydration and bleeding to anything else that causes the blood supply to the kidneys to be reduced, such as that produced by medications such as Aleve or Ibuprofen, which are the non-steroidal anti-inflammatory drugs (NSAIDs) that are used to relieve pain. Lowering of blood pressure below normal as seen in heart failure, dehydration, shock or bleeding also \reduces blood supply to the kidneys. In addition, certain medications can damage parts of the millions of structures in the kidneys which make up the filtering system (the tubules). Examples include antibiotics, X-ray dyes used to help the radiologist see your organs more easily, or anti-cancer drugs such as those containing platinum. While your doctor can correct low blood pressure, and replenish fluids and blood, and adjust antibiotic doses, the injury to the kidneys is not always predictable.

Why are kidneys so prone to injury?

The kidney is a highly functioning machine. It filters 180 liters (about 380 pints) of blood every day, to produce a urine volume of only 1.5 liters (3 pints) a day, which shows how efficient these organs are. To do this, the kidneys get about 20% of the blood coming from the heart, using up a lot of oxygen (just slightly less than the heart and more than the brain). Now you understand that the kidneys first filter and then concentrate the fluid, which causes medications to be concentrated in the kidney and damage the tubules. If oxygen is in poor supply, the damage may be increased.

Acute kidney injury can also occur from blockage of the passage of urine out of the bladder, such as stones in the draining system into the bladder (the ureters) or by blockage of the drainage system from the bladder (the urethra), by an enlarged prostate.

Recovery from acute kidney injury is possible. An operation to relieve obstruction nearly always restores kidney function (and because the tubule concentration takes a while to recover there may be a great amount of urine passed—for which you will need IV or oral fluids to keep up). Tubule damage often recovers on its own; your doctor may have to give/adjust your fluid intake, or support you by dialysis for a short period of time. Dialysis is described below. Usually only one or two dialyses is all it takes, but sometimes this may need to be continued for a while. In rare instances it may need to be prolonged forever.

The following precautions are taken for every patient to prevent acute kidney injury; medication errors and medication dosage errors are constantly being looked for and prevented. First, several medications as outlined above (NSAIDs) are avoided altogether in patients who might be at risk of developing acute kidney injury; second, all patients at risk are well hydrated before radiologic dyes are given; third, hydration is also given before anti-cancer drugs are given; and last, when possible, two or more drugs which are toxic to the kidney are not given together. Your healthcare team is especially important in kidney disease, because of the complexity of fluid balance, waste accumulation in blood, antibiotic dosing, etc. The team includes your physicians and nurses, pharmacy, nutritionist, dialysis nurses and surgeons, all of whom are concerned about your comfort, treatment and safety.

What is chronic kidney injury?

Chronic kidney injury is very common in the U.S. Chronic kidney injury has many causes, the most frequent which is diabetes, followed by high blood pressure, inflammation of the kidney (nephritis), hereditary kidney disease (polycystic kidneys), and chronic damage by certain drugs and chemicals (analgesics, lithium, etc). Because chronic kidney disease is slowly progressive, your doctor may be able to step in with treatment to control diabetes better, to control blood pressure with modern drugs, to treat the inflammation with steroids and other modern medicines, and also to prepare you for dialysis and transplantation. The first step in managing kidney disease is to recognize it—this is done by checking urine samples for protein (which should not be there at all) and checking blood for chemicals (creatinine and blood urea nitrogen) which will allow calculation of the exact amount of kidney function you have. Based on your lab test results, our hospital does an automatic calculation that serves as an alert to your physician to start looking for causes of kidney disease which can be treated.

Because the kidneys regulate chemicals and acids in the blood, chemistry tests also help your physician in detecting abnormalities in sodium, potassium, bicarbonate, calcium and phosphate for which there are specific treatments. The kidney also normally produces hormones which control anemia (erythropoietin) and bone formation (vitamin D). Chronic kidney injury is often accompanied by anemia and bone disease—fortunately in modern medicine, the hormones can be given to the patient to correct abnormalities in anemia and bone disease, and phosphate in the diet can be controlled with modern medicines. Although severe restriction of protein in the diet was felt to retard the progress of kidney disease, a large National Institutes of Health funded study showed that this was not the case. Your physician will tell you that malnutrition is never a good thing especially in dialysis patients.

If kidney function continues to decrease despite the best treatment, your physician will inform you that preparations for dialysis should be made. If you opt for hemodialysis, where the blood is cleansed of the wastes excreted by the normal kidney, you will need "permanent vascular access" for the needles to be placed in order to attach you to the dialysis machine. This means the creation of an arteriovenous fistula usually in the arm (a vein is attached to an artery with a small open connection allowing greater blood flow to the vein to create wider veins in the arm). If your surgeon does not think you have suitable blood vessels, he/she may choose to place a synthetic blood vessel between an artery and a vein in your arm. This is called an arteriovenous graft. If dialysis is needed right away, a plastic catheter will be placed in the neck under local anesthesia. To avoid infection these operations are performed in a sterile manner, and care will be taken to keep the operative site clean and free from infection.

Most patients have dialysis at a "center" but it is possible to do dialysis at home. Home hemodialysis is possible and so is peritoneal dialysis (where a catheter is placed in to the abdominal cavity to allow exchange of dialysis fluid from the outside using the lining of the abdomen to function like a dialysis membrane). Both methods require a short period of training.

If your doctor thinks you are well enough, you can avoid dialysis altogether by having what is called a "pre-emptive" transplant. This is only possible if you have somebody step forward as a donor (although most donors are family members, sometimes friends may be donors or even "buddies" on the internet can be found). If this is not possible, a transplant surgeon can assess you and place you on a "list" to wait for a kidney from a deceased donor. In order for you to become a dialysis patient you will be treated by a team which includes your physicians and nurses, nurse practitioners, social worker, pharmacy, nutritionist, dialysis nurses and surgeons, transplant coordinators, tissue typing technicians, dialysis technicians and mechanical engineers all of whom are concerned about your comfort, treatment and safety.

All precautions are taken to ensure your safety and well being. You should be on the most modern medications available, and not receiving any medications known to be harmful to the kidneys nor any other organ. Recently, modern medications for treating diabetes have been questioned in their role in increasing heart disease risk. You should discuss every medication you are taking with your kidney doctor at every visit.

What is dialysis?

"Dialysis" means the passage of chemicals through a membrane whether it is natural (peritoneal membrane) or synthetic (hemodialysis membrane). Any waste build-up is transferred across the membrane to dialysis fluid on the other side of the membrane and carried away. The chemicals transfer from blood to the dialysis fluid, and to ensure safety some chemicals required for normal body actions are not removed. This is made possible by adjusting chemicals such as sodium, potassium, calcium, and magnesium in the dialysis fluid so that at the end of treatment those chemicals are in the right concentration in your blood. All other wastes are not controlled so that you end treatment with "normalized values." To ensure safety, such as making sure that it does not contain any contaminants from the city water supply, dialysis fluid is checked every day for chemical content. Elaborate water treatment rooms in every dialysis center in the country perform these checks. Peritoneal dialysis fluid comes in sterile bags, which have the chemical content assured and adjusted individually. All patients should comply with the dialysis prescription since it has been shown that missing treatment is associated with poorer survival. It is also important to work with your nutritionist to maintain well-nourished and avoid certain foods which may be harmful to you.

Dialysis safety is our primary concern. Every dialysis center has fully-trained personnel. The procedure itself includes: aseptic insertion of needles, isolation rooms to keep you safe from infectious diseases, a clean environment, care plans to ensure treatment goals, quality improvement meetings by staff on a monthly basis, oversight of all activities by a senior management team, and grievance procedures should you not feel comfortable with any aspect of your treatment.

State government also has a "hotline" where you can make complaints about any aspect of your experience at the dialysis center. Most importantly, since there will be necessary changes in your normal schedules, you can work with social workers to get dialysis at the most convenient time for you (three times a week for 3-6 hours), and to make sure you get what you are entitled to in terms of insurance and social services. Your physician and/or nurse practitioner will see you in the center at least once a week, during which time you can have prescriptions renewed and re-evaluated. Since many patients have co-existing diseases, the center staff will guide you to see other physicians and services, which also includes seeing your kidney doctor at his/her office. We believe that the key to successful dialysis is open communication between patient, doctors, nurses, social workers and nutritionist in conjunction with other specialists.

Get to know your rights for safety and well-being—each dialysis center has them posted on the wall in the waiting area, and you can take a copy home for you and your family.

Music Therapy

Joanne V. Loewy, DA, MT-BC, LCAT

What is Music Therapy?

Music therapy is the informed use of improvised or composed music as an intervention to facilitate therapeutic change. Musical experiences and the musical relationship between a patient and a music therapist are the main dynamic factors in the therapeutic process. Physical, mental and/or spiritual issues are accessed, addressed and resolved through creating or listening to music. Verbal discourse may or may not accompany the musical experience in order to guide, interpret, enhance, identify and consolidate insights gained during the process.

Music as a healing influence in its capacity to affect health and behavior is as old as the writings of Aristotle and Plato. The 20th century discipline of music therapy officially began after World War I and World War II when musicians of all types, both amateur and professional, played for veterans in hospitals throughout the country. These patients suffered from physical and emotional trauma during and after the wars. The patients' notable physical and emotional responses to music led doctors and nurses to request the hiring of musicians by the hospitals. It was soon evident that the hospital musicians needed some prior training before entering the facility. As the demand grew for a college curriculum, the first music therapy degree program in the world began at Michigan State University in 1944. The American Music Therapy Association was founded in 1998 as a union of the National Association for Music Therapy and the American Association for Music Therapy. Today there are over 3000 music therapists in the United States and growing programs worldwide.

Music therapy is currently a creative modality of healing which is included in hundreds of hospitals throughout the world. Music therapists provide individual, group, family and community sessions for patients, families and staff. Music therapy in hospitals often addresses pain, fear or anxiety. Music experiences can assist in building resilience, trust, mastery and/or release. Music therapy is provided at the beginning of life in our maternity unit and at end of life in hospice, providing an environment of choice and dignity for patients and families who are approaching the end of life.

Since 1994, music therapy has been identified as a reimbursable service under benefits for Partial Hospitalization Programs (PHP). Falling under the heading of Activity Therapy, the interventions are not purely recreational or diversionary in nature and must be individualized and based on goals specified in the treatment plan. The current Healthcare Common Procedure Coding System (HCPCS) Code for PHP is G0176.

When should I ask for a Music Therapy Consult in the Hospital?

Music therapy referrals are typically made by members of the hospital treatment team, including doctors, nurses, social workers and clergy. Family members may also make referrals at any time by calling the music therapy department directly or through speaking with the resident or attending doctor, nurse, social worker or unit clerk.

A referral can be made to music therapy at any time and for any reason. Usually, patients who are referred for music therapy are seeking support either in areas where medicine and/or medical interventions alone are not meeting patient and/or family expectations, or to supplement and complement difficult on-going medical treatments or procedures. Music therapists may use a medical music psychotherapy approach, which means that medical aspects of care correlate with potential opportunity for music resourcing whereby music interventions are made in accordance with a holistic concept of humanistic mind-body-spirit integration. In music therapy, the cultural and intuitive domains of functioning are addressed through clinical improvisation involving the use of live music making. The active use of creativity addresses unique aspects of a person's belief systems which often present through choice of music and/or song selection.

How does music therapy work?

Each music therapist is sensitively trained to offer a variety of interventions which are based upon careful assessment of a person's preference to a particular kind of music and/or an attraction to a certain sound or instrument. The music therapy department houses hundreds of unique instruments that represent sounds from virtually all over the world.

When the assessment is complete, the information is shared with the multi-disciplinary team. Goals and specific interventions are clustered and adapted to suit the particular needs of each patient. For instance, a music therapist might accompany someone to surgery and work to relax them using a favorite Baroque piece on the violin. The therapist might move with the patient from the holding area into the operating room, providing gentle sounds entrained to the patient's breath until anesthesia has taken affect.

Patients who are experiencing pain that may or may not be having relief through pharmacological interventions may benefit from music therapy. An intervention for pain might be release oriented; the patient may discharge tension and fear through African drumming. Another patient may wish to sing an original blues about being in the hospital for an extended period. Another patient might select a favorite song or piece, and use the image of a favorite place to quietly meditate while listening to the therapist play.

How does music affect medicine?

Increasingly, we are learning that people are interested in being active participants in their own recovery. Music can significantly alter mood. It can lower and steady blood pressure or assist in helping to release tension. Music can relax or sedate, (1) it can also build resiliency. Music is intricately connected to the body and its functions; from the rhythm of the heart to the meter of the breath. We are musical beings and the timbres, tones, melodies and harmonies of music can assist in the body's capacity to balance, integrate and function in an optimal way. Music provides a humanizing element which can alter a patient's perception of a potentially frightening experience. Music can shift a seemingly sterile experience into an aesthetically pleasing environment. Figure 1, A Model of Integrative Medical Music Psychotherapy outlines the areas that medical music psychotherapy addresses. The medical aspects of care in the lower quadrant correlate to the music perspectives which are listed on the upper quadrant: Illness (medical) to Wellness (musical); Clinical objective (medical) and to Subjective response (musical).

A MODEL OF INTEGRATIVE MEDICAL MUSIC PSYCHOTHERAPY
J. Loewy & B. Scheiby, 2001

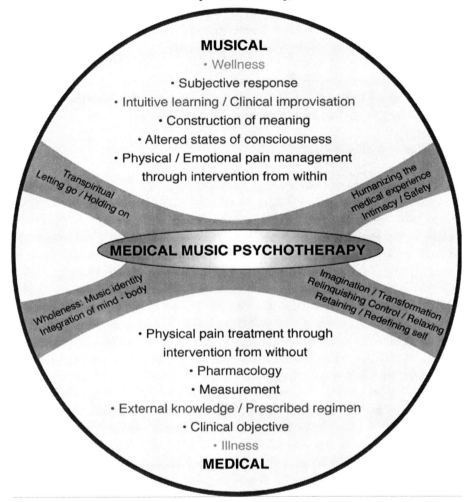

MUSICAL
- Wellness
- Subjective response
- Intuitive learning / Clinical improvisation
- Construction of meaning
- Altered states of consciousness
- Physical / Emotional pain management through intervention from within

Letting go / Holding on Transpiritual

Humanizing the medical experience Intimacy / Safety

MEDICAL MUSIC PSYCHOTHERAPY

Wholeness: Music identity Integration of mind - body

Imagination / Transformation Relinquishing Control / Relaxing Retaining / Redefining self

- Physical pain treatment through intervention from without
- Pharmacology
- Measurement
- External knowledge / Prescribed regimen
- Clinical objective
- Illness

MEDICAL

How can Music Therapy help me gain more control over my condition?

Since music exists in the context of a meter and has collaborative qualities, making music with others is an orienting and communicative activity. Unlike talking to someone, where two people take turns; one person talks while another listens; in music making one or more people can make sounds at the same time and this simultaneous experience is quite orienting especially during a procedure, or during times of pain or crisis. Music is associative and can situate one's mind and body to a particularly meaningful moment which enhances a feeling of well-being and containment.

Is there data to suggest that music therapy can help me get better faster, or reduce my need for medications?

Perioperative music has been shown to decrease stress as measured by the cortisol level and natural killer lymphocyte count.(2) Music selected by patients is more effective in reducing stress than random music.

Can music make me safer?

Being in pain and unable to sleep due to high levels of noise have been cited as significant stressors that are identified by patients, staff, and families in hospital ICUs. (3), (4), (5) High noise levels in ICUs can increase the potential for medical error. Measuring sound levels in an effort to reduce noise in hospitals, and in particular NICUs and ICUs have been the target of hospitals in recent years. (6), (7) (8). Environmental Music Therapy (EMT) has been effectively implemented at New York's Beth Israel for many years. During its inception, Stewart piloted the NICU staff to learn about their stress and perception of noise. EMT's ability to lower the noise level in the NICU was notable, and staff found that live music tailored to the environments' sounds encouraged more focus on awareness, adherence and commitment to a quieter unit. (9)

In the NICU, music and music therapy has been shown to influence weight gain, reduce needed days of hospital stays and lessen stress responses in premature infants.(10) Music therapy has also directly influenced their systolic blood pressure, heart rate, and respiratory rate. (11) Live music is particularly beneficial to preterm infants in this environment.(12) In sedating infants and toddlers for EEG (electroencephalographs), live music therapy was shown to be more effective than chloral hydrate in keeping patients asleep and since pharmacological sedation can cause respiratory depression in certain instances, music therapy may be a safer, therefore more preferable means of sedation when compared to drug agents. (13)

Music has successfully reduced pain episodes in patients with cancer (14) and at end of life (15). Music can be especially comforting to children (16) or adults who experience pain and/or high blood pressure. Music therapy can decrease a patient's perception of pain, particularly during painful procedures where anxiety and fear is elevated. (17)

Since music is a part of the average person's daily healthy life, it can be used as a positive life-evoking aesthetic modality of change when hospital care is necessary. Doctors and nurses at Beth Israel value the music therapy service and readily refer patients for music therapy as part of their patient's care plan.

We are each musical beings; from the rhythm of our heart, the timbre of our breath and in the way we integrate and orchestrate each system of the body to form an integrated alive being. Music affects the way we breathe (18) and influences our mood, endurance and physical function which can have a direct correlation to the heart and cardiac functioning. (19), (20) Music therapists work with the body's capacity to synchronize and relax which directly affects the adrenal corticosteroids and may in turn have an impact on the re-entrainment of circadian rhythms so necessary for healing. Perhaps most importantly, music can empower patients' in their capacity to gain control over their functioning, particularly when disease can feel threatening. When a person requires hospitalization, the response can be traumatic. Music therapists have studied (21) how music can reduce traumatic response. At Beth Israel, whether at the bedside, in the operating room, in the emergency room or in one of our music therapy studios, music therapy has provided a continuum of creative healing potentials and empowerment opportunities for patients, families and staff for the past 15 years.

References:

(1) Loewy, J., Hallan, C., Friedman, E., Martinez, C., Sleep/Sedation in Children Undergoing EEG Testing: A Comparison of Chloral Hydrate and Music Therapy. Journal of PeriAnesthesia Nursing, Volume 20, Issue 5, October 2005, 323-331.

(2) Leardi S, Pietroletti R, Angeloni G, Necozione S, Ranalletta G, Del Gusto B. Randomized clinical trial examining the effect of music therapy in stress response to day surgery. Br J Surg. 2007;94(8):943-947.

(3) Hweidi, IM, Psychological consequences associated with intensive care treatment. Trauma. 2007; 9: 95-102.

(4) So, H.M. & Chan, D.S. Perception of stressors by patients and nurses of critical care units in Hong Kong. Int. J. Nurs. Stud., 2004, 41, 77-84

(5) Russell, S. An exploratory study of patient' perceptions, memories, and experiences of an intensive care unit. Journal of Advanced Nursing, 1999, 29 (4), 783-791.

(6) Evans, J.B. & Philbin, M.K. Facility and operations planning for quiet hospital nurseries. Journal of Perinatology, Dec 2000, S105-12.

(7) Gray, L. & Philbin, M.K. Measuring sound in hospital nurseries. Journal of Perinatology, Dec 2000, S100-4.

(8) Cabrera, I.N. and Lee, M.H.M. Reducing noise pollution in the hospital setting by establishing a department of sound: a survey of recent research on the effects of noise and music in health care. Preventive Medicine, 2000, 30, 339-345.

(9)   Stewart, K. & Schneider, S., Environmental Music Therapy. In Loewy J. V. (Ed) Music therapy in the NICU. 2000, NY, NY: Satchnote Armstrong Press, 85-1—ISBN 978-0-980355-1-0.

(10)   Caine, J. The effects of music on the selected stress behaviors, weight, caloric and formula intake, and length of hospital stay of premature and low birth weight neonates in a newborn intensive care unit. Journal of Music Therapy, 1992, 28(4), 180-192.

(11)   Lorch, C., Lorch, V., Diefendorf, A., & Earl, P., Effect of stimulative and sedative music on systolic blood pressure, heart rate, and respiratory rate in premature infants. Journal of Music Therapy, 1994, 31(2), 105-118.

(12)   Arnon, S., Shapsa, A., Forman, L., Regev, R., Bauer, S., Litmanovitz, I., & Dolfin, T.Live music is beneficial to preterm infants in the neonatal intensive care unit environment. Birth, 2006, 33(2), 131-136.

(13)   Loewy, J., Hallan, C., Friedman, E., Martinez, C., Sleep/Sedation in Children Undergoing EEG Testing: A Comparison of Chloral Hydrate and Music Therapy. American Journal of Electroneurodiagnostic Technology, 46, No.4, 2006, 343-355.

(14)   Loewy, J. Music Therapy, in Barraclough, J. (Ed), Enhancing Cancer Care: Complementary therapy and support. London, England: Oxford University press. 2007, ISBN13: 9780199297559ISBN10: 019929755X

(15)   Dileo, C. & Loewy, J. Music Therapy at the End of Life. 2004, Cherry Hill, NJ: Jeffrey Books ISBN 9780980135503.

(16)   Loewy, J. Music therapy pediatric pain management: Assessing and attending to the sounds of hurt, fear and anxiety, in Music Therapy in Pediatric Pain, Loewy (Ed). 1997, Cherry Hill, N.J.: Jeffrey Books.

(17)   Malone, A. B., The effects of live music on the distress of pediatric patients receiving intravenous starts, venipunctures, injections, and heel sticks. Journal of Music Therapy, 1996, 33, 19-33.

(18)   Azoulay, R. & Loewy, J. (In-Press), Music, the Breath & Health: Advances in Integrative Music Therapy, 2008, New York, NY: Satchnote Armstrong Press.

(19)   MacNay, S. K. The influence of preferred music on the perceived exertion, mood, and time estimation scores of patients participating in a cardiac rehabilitation exercise program. Music Therapy Perspectives, 1995, 13, 91-96.

(20)   Rider, M., Floyd, J. W., & Kirkpatrick, J. The effect of music, imagery, and relaxation on adrenal corticosteroids and the re-entrainment of circadian rhythms. Journal of Music Therapy, 1985, 22, 46-58.

(21)   Loewy, J & Stewart, K. Mass trauma and violence: Helping families and children cope. In Webb, Nancy Boyd (Ed.). Music Therapy to Help Traumatized Children and Caregivers, 2004, NY, NY: Guildford Press, 191-215. ISBN 1572309768.

Orthopedic Surgery

Peter D. McCann, M.D.

In recent years, orthopedic surgery has become one of the fastest growing surgical fields. Several factors account for this: a dramatic improvement in surgical techniques, especially with regards to joint replacement surgery and arthroscopic surgery; and our population (both young and old) is ever more active, leading to increased numbers of acute injuries as well as developing degenerative or "wear and tear" damage to joints and tendons requiring reconstructive surgery in years hence. If you need an orthopedic procedure, you obviously wish to have the best outcome in the safest environment. I have found in my own practice as an orthopedic surgeon, specializing in shoulder surgery for the past 23-years, that preparation preoperatively is one of the most important aspects in obtaining a safe and excellent outcome following your surgery. I believe that preparation for one's surgery can be divided into two areas: choosing your surgeon and hospital (usually inseparable), and planning for your recovery.

How should I choose my Orthopedic Surgeon?

Most patients choose their surgeon through recommendations from their family doctor or a friend or a relative who had similar surgery. Although this method lacks a "scientific" assessment of quality, it is a system that has served most of us extremely well over the years. It is a simple system that, frankly, makes sense. Family doctors whose patients have received excellent care from a treating orthopedic surgeon and have had successful outcomes, will continue to recommend that orthopedic surgeon. Similarly, friends or relatives who have had excellent outcomes following treatment with a particular surgeon also are a sensible "sources" for choosing your doctor in the "medical marketplace". Such recommendations are based on "good results" and are an excellent, though not "objective" measure of quality of care.

However, in coming years, I believe that objective quality information on surgeon practices will be available on the internet, and that choosing one's surgeon based on reliable quality outcomes (complication rate, mortality, infection rate, etc . . . .) will become more commonplace. One example of quality assessment of surgeon practices is offered by the healthcare assessment company, HealthGrades, viewable on their website, *www.healthgrades.com*.

How should I Choose my Hospital?

Many surgeons operate at a single institution and, consequently, once you have chosen your surgeon, you have effectively chosen your hospital as well. This is both a logical and "safe" practice. As a patient, you want your surgeon to work with a consistent and familiar team. "Practice" DOES make "perfect!" and there is no advantage for a surgeon to operate at various hospitals within the same region. Depending on the nature of your surgical procedure, you will have your surgery on an ambulatory basis (that is, you are discharged from the hospital on the same day of your surgery) or you will be admitted to the hospital for post-operative care. The percentage of ambulatory procedures has increased dramatically in recent years owing to improvements in both surgical (more arthroscopic equipment) and anesthetic techniques (i.e. more regional anesthesia). These days, the only orthopedic operations that require hospitalization are the major reconstructive spine and joint replacement surgeries and major long bone fractures such as hip fractures. Ratings on the quality of hospital care can be reviewed on the Medicare website *www.cms.hhs/gov*

What Do I Need to Do to Prepare for my Surgery?

Once you have chosen your surgeon, the process of preparation begins. As the operating surgeon, I believe that it is my obligation to educate each of my patients, and you should expect the same of your surgeon. Following obtaining a history and physical examination, your surgeon should discuss with you the following essential points: understand your diagnosis and be able to explain it in everyday terms; review the various options of treatment, both operative and non-operative; describe both the nature of the surgical procedure in terms you understand and the aftercare required for your recovery; discuss the expected outcome; and, finally, appreciate the risks and possible complications associated with your surgical procedure. This discussion in the surgeon's office prior to any surgical procedure is, I believe, the most important aspect in your preparation. The more you understand about your condition and the treatment, the better you will be able to participate in the recovery to ensure the best and safest outcome.

For an excellent perspective on the risks of surgery, I highly recommend the book "Complications" by Atul Gawande, MD. (1).

What should I expect when I am in the Hospital?

If your surgery requires in hospital care, you will interact with many individuals during your hospitalization. You will discover that running a hospital and providing high quality care requires many staff members!

After your surgery and when you are on the hospital floor, your nurses and nurses' aids will be providing your postoperative care. The surgeon in charge of your care, usually referred to as the attending doctor, should see you daily following your surgery. Every surgeon needs help to provide all the care you require while in the hospital, and these "helpers" may include physician assistants, surgical interns and residents, surgical fellows, and nurse practitioners. You should expect that any member of your doctor's surgical team should introduce him or herself upon first meeting and explain their relationship with the attending surgeon. This not only is courteous, but also is essential for you to understand the relationship of the healthcare provider to your surgeon.

Very often, this surgical team will be involved in assisting your surgeon during your operation, and you should be sure to review with your doctor the extent of involvement of his or her assistants and gain the assurance of your surgeon that he or she will be performing the principal and most important aspects of your surgery. Very often the routine portions of the surgery (such as closing the wound and suturing the skin) are performed by surgical assistants and, in my experience, the assistants who perform the wound closures often do so with much better cosmetic results than I would myself since my assistants perform this portion of the procedure much more frequently than I do.

Questions always come up during your hospital stay, and you should by all means ask members of the nursing staff or surgical team any question that comes to mind. Members of the surgical team are well qualified to answer routine questions, and if there are any issues that the surgical team is unable to address, your attending doctor will. The surgical team can answer the vast majority of questions that you may have regarding your surgery and recovery, but you should also feel free to question your attending surgeon directly during his or her daily rounds.

What should I expect in preparing for discharge from the Hospital?

Discharge from the hospital following your surgery is always a cause for concern and apprehension. I have found that the best way to minimize any nervousness regarding discharge is to be very clear with my patients preoperatively the conditions that must be met for them to go home. Simply put, this requires that you be independent with "activities of daily living", that is you are mobile enough to get out of bed, walk to the bathroom, clean yourself in the bathroom, and be able to dress yourself with minimal assistance, as well as being able to manage your pain with oral medication.

The most important aspect of planning your discharge however, begins with your initial consultation with your treating surgeon in the office. Your surgeon should advise you as to which day would be the usual anticipated discharge date, and share with you the information required for you to manage at home upon discharge. For patients who will not gain sufficient independence to be discharged home at the completion of their hospitalization, transfer to either an acute rehabilitation facility or a skilled nursing facility is an option. These details should be reviewed with your operating surgeon prior to your surgery, and be determined well before your hospitalization.

In summary, I have found that the best way for patients to get the best quality of healthcare is to be an active participant in this process. The most important thing for you to do as a patient is to be prepared, understand the nature of your surgery, and anticipate what will occur while you are in the hospital. My final bit of advice is to understand that you can never be 100% prepared and that questions will arise during your hospitalization. When such questions arise, engage your healthcare team and obtain the information that you require to ensure the best and safest possible outcome following your surgery.

Other sources that you might consider for reviewing your orthopedic care include reviewing the website of your treating physician if available, as well as our professional society website, *www.AAOS.com*

References:

1. Gawande, A. Complications—A Surgeon's Notes on an Imperfect Science. New York, NY: Picador, Henry Holt and Company, 2002.

Palliative Care and Hospice

Russell Portenoy, M.D.

What is "palliative care"?

Patients and families may be confused about the term "palliative care" or other terms that are sometimes used at the same time, including "hospice" and "end-of-life care". This confusion is not surprising because the practice of palliative care in the United States has changed a great deal in recent years.

Palliative care is not the same as hospice or end-of-life care. Palliative care is both an *approach* to the treatment of patients and their families (a model of care) and a *specific medical discipline*. In just a few countries, including the United States, palliative care has become a formal medical subspecialty and doctors who want to be specialists can obtain advanced training and then take an examination to become Board Certified.

Palliative care can be defined as ***an approach to the treatment of patients with any type of serious or life-threatening illness that attempts to help the patient, and his or her family, maintain a good quality of life and reduce the sources of suffering throughout the course of the illness.***

According to an important document created by the "National Consensus Project for Best Practices in Palliative Care," the *core elements* of palliative care include the following:

- **Patient populations.** The patients appropriate for palliative care include those of all ages who are experiencing a serious or life-threatening illness, such as cancer, HIV/AIDS, Alzheimer's disease or other neurodegenerative disease, congestive heart failure, chronic obstructive pulmonary disease, cirrhosis, or advanced kidney disease.
- **Patient- and family-centered care**. Palliative care considers the patient and the family as the "unit of care" and always considers the

goals and preferences of the patient and family in developing a plan of care. The family is defined by the patient.

- **Timing of palliative care.** Palliative care should be available from the time of diagnosis through cure, or until death and into the family's period of mourning.
- **Comprehensive care.** To provide competent palliative care, health care professionals must address a broad array of concerns that may influence physical, psychological, social and spiritual well being.
- **Interdisciplinary team.** Palliative care should be on the "radar screen" of every health professional involved with a patient who has a serous illness. Patients who have complex needs ideally should have access to specialists in palliative care. *Specialist palliative care* always involves a team that includes, at minimum, a physician, a nurse, a social worker, and a pastoral care provider; the team also may include volunteers, a bereavement coordinator, a psychologist, a pharmacist, nursing assistants or home attendants, a dietitian, or others.
- **Attention to relief of suffering.** Palliative care seeks to maintain a good quality of life and reduce suffering by preventing and relieving the many and various burdens imposed by diseases and their treatments.
- **Communication skills.** Good palliative care emphasizes communication with patients and families about sensitive issues that arise in the setting of advanced illness, such as the setting of treatment goals, concerns that surround the possibility of dying, and planning for decisions if the patient can no longer make decisions.
- **Skill in care of the dying and the bereaved.** Palliative care specialists work as a team to help patients and families through the difficult period just before death, to try to ensure that the death is peaceful, dignified, devoid of distress, and consistent with the values and desires of the patient. Palliative care also recognizes the need to support families during the period after the death.
- **Continuity of care across settings.** Patients with serious illnesses often receive care in many sites, including home, hospital (both outpatient and inpatient), emergency department, and nursing home. Good palliative care strives to coordinate treatments across all these sites to prevent crises and reduce unnecessary transfers.
- **Equitable access.** Specialists in palliative care believe that comprehensive, patient and family-centered palliative care should be available to all ages and patient populations, whatever the diagnosis, setting of care, insurance coverage or other characteristics. The goal for the United States is for all professionals to incorporate the core elements of palliative care into the management of appropriate patients, and at the same time, provide access to a specialist team for any patient or family who could benefit.

- **Quality improvement.** Palliative care services should be committed to excellence and high quality of care.

What is hospice and how is it different than palliative care?

In the United States, hospice is a health care system supported by government insurance (Medicare or Medicaid) and usually by private insurers as well. This system was established more than two decades ago to provide comprehensive palliative care to patients with advanced illnesses and their families. There are now more than 4000 hospice agencies in the United States, which together provide care to more than one million patients and families each year. A large majority of those who access hospice care do so under the Medicare or Medicaid hospice benefit, which is an entitlement like Social Security. This benefit provides a *home care program* with access to a specialist palliative care team (physician, nurse, social worker and chaplain) and also pays the costs of other services, drugs and other needs related to the terminal illness. *It must be emphasized that hospice is not a place and is not only concerned with dying.* It is a program of services that should be used by those with advanced illness to achieve the goals of palliative care: maintaining quality of life and preventing or relieving the suffering related to the burden of the illness.

Although some specialist palliative care teams also work in home care, most of these teams are situated in hospitals or in nursing homes. Hospital-based specialist palliative care services usually refer appropriate patients to hospice programs to gain access to benefits and provide services at home.

In the hospital, what should patients expect from a palliative care service?

About half of the hospitals in the United States now have some kind of a team to provide specialist palliative care. These teams try to follow the core elements of palliative care. More specifically, they are available to be consulted when patients with serious or life-threatening illnesses, or their families, develop complex or challenging problems that complicate care or increase suffering. The major areas of concern (also called the "domains") of specialist palliative care include:

- **Structure and processes of care.** If a palliative care team is consulted in the hospital, the patient and family should meet an interdisciplinary group of professionals who will try to work with the primary physician, the floor nurses and social worker, and others to develop a palliative plan of care. This may involve the treatment of symptoms or other problems, or assistance with discharge planning; it may include referral to a palliative care unit in the hospital or referral on discharge to a home care agency or a local hospice program if the patient is eligible for these services.

- **Physical aspects of care.** The palliative care team is expert in pain and symptom control and also is concerned with addressing other physical concerns, such as the management of complications like skin ulcers and assistance in maintaining function.
- **Psychological and psychiatric aspects of care.** The palliative team will assess the patient and family for problems like anxiety and depression or grief, and assist in the management of these conditions. It is expert in dealing with the problem of delirium, particularly the confusion that may occur at the end of life.
- **Social aspects of care.** The team is concerned with the well being of the family and will try to help the patient maintain positive relationships within the family and with friends. The team also may try to help the patient deal with problems that undermine intimacy with a loved one.
- **Spiritual, religious and existential aspects of care.** The palliative care team should assess the patient and family for the occurrence of distress associated with spiritual concerns and the possibility that spiritual or religious care can be beneficial in trying to adapt to the losses associated with a serious illness. In the hospital, a chaplain associated with the palliative care team may try to help with acute needs or request permission to contact clergy in the community to try to assist a patient or the family after discharge from the hospital.
- **Cultural aspects of care.** Palliative care teams recognize that there is extraordinary diversity among patients and families and referral to a palliative care team should ensure that care is culturally-sensitive.
- **Care of the imminently dying patient.** Specialists in palliative care can provide expert care during the period immediately before and after a death. These times often are challenging, and as a result, the palliative care team often is consulted when death is perceived to be imminent. During this time, members of the team ensure that the patient is comfortable, other needs are met, and the family is supported.
- **Ethical and legal aspects of care.** The care of patients with serious illnesses always should be founded on ethical decision making. Some of the most difficult issues are encountered when the illness is advanced. In some cases, a consultation to the palliative care team may be able to clarify key issues and ensure that treatment decisions are medically appropriate and reflect the goals of care and the values of the patient and family.

How do I know when I should seek a palliative care consult?

A patient or a member of the family may perceive that a palliative care consultation may be helpful. If the patient has a serious or life-threatening illness, and there is distress related to poorly controlled symptoms, psychological problems, family issues, or other potential sources of suffering, the palliative care team may be able to help. If planning for care after discharge from the hospital is complicated, the palliative care team may be able to provide some insights about home care services. Finally, if the doctors have indicated that death may occur during this admission to the hospital, referral to the palliative care team may ensure that professionals are available who have a special expertise in managing the problems that occur at the end of life.

Should I wait for my doctor to offer a palliative care consultation, or should I request it?

Palliative care is a very young specialty in the United States. Although it is remarkable to observe, it is a reality that many physicians and other professionals do not yet know about specialist palliative care. Even more amazing, it is common for these professionals to have incorrect information about palliative care or hospice. It is not uncommon, for example, for patients or families to hear from their physicians that palliative care is for the dying, hospice is a place and not a program, or that the expertise of palliative care specialists (such as the skills in pain and symptom control) can be obtained through multiple consultations with other doctors. Because misconceptions are so common among health professionals, patients and families *must* be willing to request (and even *demand*) a palliative care consultation if there is a chance that a specialist palliative care team can help relieve distress.

References or Resources for Palliative Care

www.StopPain.org—the website for the Department of Pain Medicine and Palliative Care at Beth Israel Medical Center.

www.nationalconsensusproject.org/Guideline.pdf—a website that describes the clinical practice guideline developed by the National Consensus Project for Best Practices in Palliative Care.

www.growthhouse.org—an informational website for patients and others that describes many aspects of palliative care.

www.nhpco.org—the official website for the National Hospice and Palliative Care Organization, which provides a great deal of information to patients and families about hospice and palliative care.

www.grievingcenter.org—a website about grief and bereavement.

Care of the Pediatric Patient

Edward Conway, M.D.

There are approximately three million infants, children and adolescents hospitalized annually in the United States. Although there is a recent trend for fewer admissions for pediatric aged patients, those who are admitted are sicker and will require longer hospital stays. There are twice as many children in the 0-4 year old group admitted compared with those in the 5-14 year old group. [1] There are many different types of hospitals where your child may be admitted and these include community, university, county, children's and others. Different hospitals may have different age requirements but many admit pediatric aged patients up to the age of 16 and some through 21 years depending on their capabilities and areas of expertise. Pediatric aged patients are usually divided as follows: infants are usually considered up to 1 year of age, children 2-12 years of age and adolescents 13-18 years. The major possible reasons for your child needing to be admitted are for an acute illnesses (e.g. respiratory illness, pneumonia, dehydration, gastroenteritis) or injury (head trauma, significant extremity fracture), exacerbations of existing chronic illness (asthma, diabetes, seizures. sickle cell disease), planned medical or surgical admissions and possibly PICU admissions for diseases or injuries which result in your child being in an unstable critical condition. You child's pediatrician or primary care provider should be your first resource to ensure your child gets the appropriate care and admitted to the hospital best suited to handle your child's medical or surgical issue(s). Once your child is admitted to the hospital the coordination and oversight of their care may be provided by either your primary care provider or by another physician, but you want to be sure "there is a captain of the ship" managing your child's care. You want to know who they are and how you can contact them.

How do I select a high quality hospital for my child?

In today's electronic age and with rapid access to the internet one is just a few clicks away from obtaining most information that will be helpful. You can quickly log on to the hospitals' web site and quickly browse their website for specific information and then find their Pediatric site. It will usually give you a brief overview and allow you to look at the services and types of physicians that will be available to care for your child. Another way to determine if the hospital is appropriate for a pediatric admission is to know if it is approved by the Joint Commission. This is an organization which provides oversight and accreditation and if accredited the institution will have met standards demonstrating the provision of developmentally appropriate care, effective communication for patient education, consideration of safety issues, and provide age-appropriate environments and assessment of patients. [1]

Your child's primary care physician/pediatrician will have admitting privileges at one or more hospitals where he/she is credentialed to admit and render care to their patients. They will be a primary resource for many of your questions and concerns. You will also have access to other families in the practice where your child is cared for. You can ask other families their experiences with the various hospitals and services they provide. One must be cautious as some of those families may have a love or hate of a particular institution which is not based on what will be important for you and your child!

In order for a physician to be credentialed to admit and care for patients in the hospital they must undergo the following: 1) assessment of professional and personal background, 2) assignment of privileges appropriate for their clinical training and experience, 3) ongoing monitoring of professional activity and 4) periodic (every two years) reappointment to the Hospital's Medical Staff based on the above in conjunction with objectively monitored on-going performance. A privilege is a specific permission by the hospital for an individual practitioner to perform diagnostic or therapeutic procedures or other patient care services within well-defined limits (based on training and experience). [2] In addition to being on various Hospital Staff(s) your primary care physician/pediatrician should belong to societies associated with their particular area of expertise. Many pediatricians have the initials FAAP following their name and this stands for Fellow of the American Academy of Pediatrics. Approximately 60,000 pediatricians in the United States currently have earned this distinction. It attests that they have trained in an approved pediatric training program and successfully passed their certifying examination in general pediatrics. They are then also called board-certified pediatricians and have made an ongoing commitment to lifelong learning and advocacy for children. In order to maintain the FAAP designation the pediatrician must continue to study and attend courses yearly (also called continuing medical education), maintain their state licensure, and pass another examination every seven years (this will change to every 10 years in 2010).

What can I expect when my child is hospitalized?

As mentioned previously the care of hospitalized children has become increasingly complex. Your child may have a condition that warrants involvement of other physicians which may include medical and or surgical sub specialists. Technology dependent children (e.g. those on home ventilation, tracheotomies, G-tubes, central venous access devices, ventriculoperitoneal shunts, etc . . .) present a specific set of challenges. They may need in addition to the primary care attending, other consultants to care for them. These children will require an entire team of pediatric specialists which may include in addition to the physicians, nurses, social workers, chaplains, child life, occupational and physical therapists, nutritionist, respiratory therapists, music therapists and many others.

Once the decision has been made to admit your child (from the clinic, your physician's office, or the emergency department) it is natural that your anxiety level will rise. It is essential that upon admission a complete evaluation be performed and this will include the reason why your child is being admitted and the events surrounding this admission (history of present illness HPI), your child's past medical history (PMH), a review of organ systems where you will be asked specific questions about everything from head, eyes, ears, nose, mouth, glands, neck, chest, lungs, heart, abdomen, genitalia, hips, legs, feet etc . . ., history of immunizations (if you have the card it is best to always bring that with you), an assessment of growth and development, pain assessment, and a social history with a focus on behavioral and emotional issues. [3] Your child will then be examined by both the medical and nursing staff. Other staff members may visit to perform an assessment which may include social work and nutritional services. Your child may need blood tests, an intravenous line may need to be inserted and imaging studies may be required. It is important that you ask why the tests are being performed and that you be notified when the results are available. If your child has a significant past medical history it is best if you bring whatever medical documentation you have to the hospital to help the team understand your child's particular problem. There are many different types of forms available but the American Academy of Pediatrics has one called the Emergency Information Form for Children with Special Needs which is excellent, easy to complete and very helpful. A copy of this form is easily downloaded from the AAP website at (www.aap.org). The hospital medical staff is cognizant of how tedious it may be to the parents of a child with a complex medical/surgical problem to repeat the history and events surrounding the admission more than once, however it is essential that the medical staff (particularly if they have not cared for your child previously) review all the information to provide the best possible care for your child. Be sure to tell the physicians/medical staff what medications your child is taking and what allergies your child may have. It is helpful to know if your child has had unusual reactions to medications in the past and their response to pain and prior surgical procedures. Also remember that your child's admission is a two way street and it is important that you ask the staff any questions and voice any concerns you may have. At our hospital there are white boards in each room. These are simply dry marker boards where our staff will ask the patient and parents what we can do to make your hospital stay the best possible one. These boards are helpful as they allow communication between family and staff. They are updated daily. Common comments we have seen include: make the stay pain free, let us sleep, please knock, please explain why we need this test, please give us the result of the test as soon as you have it, etc . . . The children and adolescents enjoy putting their comment on the boards as well and these range from those cited above to requests for a particular DVD, no blood tests, a particular video-game or pizza! Again it allows for the patient to have some control but most importantly engenders communication between the patient, family and staff.

The medical team will usually round twice a day. The first time is in the morning (usually 7-10 AM) when the physician, nurses and many other team members will review your child's admission information data, examine your child, review pertinent tests that were performed and then make a plan for the day. It is a good time to catch the physicians/nurses when they are finished rounding so that they can discuss the plans for your child for the day. Evening sign-out rounds occur later in the day (4-6 PM) and the progress of your child for that day is discussed and plans are made for the night to anticipate what your child may need (e.g. blood tests, imaging studies (x-rays, CTs, MRIs, etc). This is again another good time to check in with the medical team.

Who will be members of my child's healthcare team?

There will be a physician assigned to your child's care and it may or may not be your child's primary care provider. There are physicians called Hospitalists who provide in-house care for hospitalized patients and they can be found in many hospitals currently. Other members of the medical team that may provide direct medical care to your child may include nurse practitioners (NPs) and physician assistants (PAs). An NP is a registered nurse with advanced education and clinical training beyond the usual 2 to 4 years of basic nursing education required for state nursing licensure. The additional training may be through a certificate program or a master's degree program. A PA is registered by the state after 2 or more years of undergraduate education followed by 9 to 12 months of preclinical didactic studies and 9 to 15 months of physician-supervised clinical education. [4] Other physicians that may be involved in the care of your child include pediatric and adult sub specialists and surgeons along with medical students, residents and fellows. In the event that a patient is admitted to an adult service or if the primary physician does not have sufficient pediatric experience, or if the patient has complex medical or psychosocial problems, age ≤ 14 years or a weight of ≤ 40kg it is recommended that a pediatric consultation be obtained.

Pediatric sub specialists that may be consulted include allergy, adolescent medicine, cardiology, developmental pediatrics, endocrinology, emergency medicine, gastrointestinal physicians, genetics, hematology, infectious disease, neurology, nephrology, psychiatry, psychology, radiology, rheumatology, and sports medicine. The reader is referred to the AAP website at *aap.org* for particular descriptions of the diseases these experts manage and their qualification. Surgical subspecialties include pediatric surgery, otolaryngology (ear, nose and throat experts), ophthalmology (eye), orthopedics (bone), neurosurgery (brain and spinal cord), plastic surgery and urology. The key to a successful hospitalization is communication between the team and with the parents and patient (if age appropriate) in an on-going open-ended dialogue.

Many hospitals will have a Child Life Program. Child life practitioners provide developmentally appropriate play therapy, preoperative and postoperative psychological preparation and help children to develop coping skills and provide family support during this very trying period. Other members of the team may include music therapists and some hospitals will provide pet therapy.

Hospitals that have made the commitment to care for pediatric patients will usually adhere to what has been termed Family Centered Care. This is defined as care that is accessible, continuing and comprehensive, family centered, coordinated, compassionate and culturally sensitive and effective. [5]

Will my child be separated from other adult patients?

Yes, pediatric patients are admitted to a separate ward than their adult counterparts. Pediatric patients may be grouped by age (e.g. infants, children and adolescents segregated by age) or all pediatric aged patients may be admitted to a single unit based on bed availability and particular hospital policy and procedures. As mentioned previously each hospital will have its own age cutoffs for admission to a particular ward/service. Pediatrics is usually considered less than 14 years, however many larger community hospitals and children's hospitals will admit up until the patient's 21st birthday. The important concept is that the pediatric aged patients be housed together to allow for the delivery of age/developmental specific care for your child.

Will I or my family be allowed to stay with my child?

Each hospital has its own visiting policy. Many children's hospitals and larger community based hospitals will allow one parent to sleep at the bedside of the patient but one needs to be aware that not all hospitals can accommodate this request. It is important that anyone with a fever, rash or suspected respiratory illness not visit the patient while they are in the hospital as this will impose a risk of a potential infectious exposure to the patient. It is also important to recognize that patients, and their families, need to rest and to ensure that they get proper amounts of sleep.

How do we assure that the staff knows how to dose the medications correctly for children?

Errors associated with medications are believed to be the most common type of medical error and the incidence is about three times that of errors occurring in adult patients. [6] Children are more prone because most medications used in their care are formulated and packaged for adults, most health care settings are based on the needs of adults, young sick infants and children are less able to tolerate a medication error due to their immature and still developing kidney, liver and immune functions and lastly children are not able to communicate to their caretakers adverse effects the meds may be causing. The Joint Commision and many other organizations have made patient safety their number one concern and have implemented many strict risk reduction strategies to prevent medication errors in children so again, if the hospital where your child is admitted is certified by The Joint Commission, they had to demonstrate that all of the safety strategies are in place.

Examples of these guidelines include: a pediatric formulary system with policy for drug evaluation exists, limit the number of concentrations and does strengths of high alert medications to the minimum needed to provide safe care, use oral syringes to administer oral medications, assign a practitioner trained in pediatrics to any committee that is responsible for the oversight of medication management, provide dose calculation sheets for each pediatric critical care patient and create pediatric satellite pharmacies and have a pediatric pharmacist available or on-call at all times. Since weight is used to calculate most dosing, all pediatric patients should be weighed in kilograms' at the time of admission or within four hours of admission in an emergency situation. Kilograms should be the standard nomenclature for weight on prescriptions, medical records and staff communications. Lastly in the event that a medication error does occur, the hospital must perform a root cause analysis (which is an extensive review of all the details involved in what caused the error) and then the hospital must develop and implement a corrective action plan which is to be monitored to ensure that it is effective. As a parent the most important way you can prevent medical errors is to be a part of your child's health care team. You should be involved in every decision that is made about your child's care. Be sure to tell the physicians all of the medications your child is taking, and any allergic reactions they may have experienced. When you are discharged from the hospital be sure you can read the prescription, ask for information about the medication from the pharmacy and if you have any questions ask them! You can always check with your physician and/or nurse before you leave. They will perform a medicine reconciliation which is where they review what meds your child came in on and what meds they are being discharged to home with. If there are any discrepancies or questions this is an excellent time to discuss them.

What should I do if I have a question or concern about my child's care?

As noted above the most important thing you can do is to be an active member of your child's healthcare team. Get involved and ask questions. Many different healthcare providers will interact with you and your child and you should feel comfortable asking any of them your questions. **Communication** is the key to a successful hospitalization. The primary attending for your child will be directing the healthcare team with input from many possible health care providers. It will be his/her job to decide to implement (or not) recommendations from the various sub specialists that may be involved as well as decision making for further testing and evaluation of your child. It is important that you understand what is being done and why. There is an old adage that if someone cannot explain something they don't understand it themselves!

When do I need to consider a specialized Children's Hospital?

Infants and children with major congenital anomalies (brain, heart, lungs, liver etc.), malignancies, transplants, major trauma and severe chronic illnesses should be managed by pediatric medical and surgical specialists at pediatric referral centers. These centers can provide expertise in many areas including the medical and surgical specialties, pediatric radiology, pediatric anesthesiology, pediatric pathology and pediatric intensive care. The optimal management of the child with complex problems, chronic illness, or disabilities requires coordination, communication and cooperation of the pediatric surgical specialist with your child's primary care pediatrician or physician. [7]

Resources for children and their parents in the hospital.

Many hospitals will give you a welcome packet that will contain much valuable information concerning how the Pediatric Unit operates, visiting policies, other specific hospital policies, a copy of the patient bill of rights and other useful information. They may also contain information on local hotels, stores, restaurants, take-out and delivery menus, laundromats, movie rental stores to cite a few examples. They also usually contain important phone numbers to allow you to contact members of your child's team and to directly call the hospital's units. As a parent and advocate for your child you should feel free to ask questions and start a dialogue with all members of your child's team.

If my child is sick is it better to be seen in a Pediatric Emergency Department than an adult ED?

It is unusual for infants and children to become seriously ill without warning. If you are concerned you should immediately call your child's primary care provider/pediatrician. An emergency is defined as a feeling that there is an injury or illness imminently endangering your child's health. If the injury or illness is severe and you think it may endanger your child's life then immediately call 911 (or your local emergency number). If you think that your child may have ingested a poison or someone else's medication you should call a poison control center even if the child does not have any immediate signs or symptoms. (1-800-222-1222).

A recent study demonstrated that 89% of pediatric emergency visits occur in non-children's hospitals and many occur in fact in emergency departments that do not see many pediatric visits per year (defined as less than 7000 visits/year). The vast majority of pediatric visits occur in emergency departments shared with adult patients and children were seen in a separate area in only 4% of the EDs in the study. [8] Emergency Departments with a high pediatric volume and facilities with physician and nursing coordinators specifically for pediatrics were better prepared to care for children. There are 13 specific ED policies that were published by the American Academy of Pediatrics (AAP) and the American College of Medicine (ACEP) for emergency departments to address the specific needs of children. Emergency departments that were aware of these policies were better prepared to care for children. The 13 ED policies include: child maltreatment, informed consent, sedation and analgesia, illness and injury triage, immunization status, transfers necessary for definitive care, death in the ED, mental health emergencies, disaster plan, do-not-resuscitate orders, communication with patient's primary health care provider, physical restraint of pediatric patients and family issues/family presence. As a parent reading the above list it is obvious that the best ED for your child to be evaluated in should have all of these policies in place. It is evidence that there is a commitment to Pediatrics as well as contingency plans for transfer in the event that the particular hospital where your child is being seen is unable to provide the in-patient or Pediatric Critical Care that your child may require. They will ensure safe transportation from their facility to one with the proper equipment and physician/nursing personnel which your child requires.

CONCLUSIONS

As a result of the Institute of Medicine's 2001 report *Crossing the Quality Chasm: A New Health System for the 21ˢᵗ Century*, there has been an emphasis on the need to ensure the involvement of patients in their own health care decisions, to better inform patents of treatment options, and to improve patients' and families' access to information. [9] These recommendations are also intrinsic to family centered practice. You want to seek a hospital that supports the core principles of family-centered care. Family-centered care embraces collaborative relationships between patients, families, physicians, nurses, and other professionals for the planning, delivery, and evaluation of health care as well as in the education of health care professionals. A summary of these core principles are as follows: respecting each child and their family; honoring racial, ethnic, cultural and socioeconomic diversity; recognizing and building on the strengths of each child and family; supporting and facilitation of choice about approaches to care, ensuring flexibility in organizational policies; sharing unbiased information and providing or ensuring formal and informal support for the child and parent(s) and/or guardian(s) during pregnancy, childbirth, infancy, childhood, adolescence, and young adulthood; collaborating with families and empowering each child and family to discover their own strengths, build confidence, and make choices and decisions about their health. [5]

Remember that the best thing you can do for your child during a hospital admission is to advocate for them and keep the lines of communication open. We as physicians are privileged to care for your children and we aim to earn your trust. At our hospital every infant, child and adolescent is treated as if they were our own child and if my children were admitted to a hospital I would expect no less, nor should you.

REFERENCES

1) American Academy of Pediatrics. Committee on Hospital Care. Child Life Services. Pediatrics. 2006:118:1757-1763.

2) American Academy of Pediatrics. O'Connor ME and the Committee on Hospital Care. Medical Staff Appointment and Delineation of Pediatric Privileges in Hospitals. Pediatrics. 2002;110:414-418.

3) American Academy of Pediatrics. Percelay JM and the Committee on Hospital Care. Physician's Roles in Coordinating Care of Hospitalized Children. Pediatrics. 2003;111:707-709.

4) American Academy of Pediatrics. Committee on Hospital Care. The Role of Nurse Practitioner and Physician Assistant in the Care of Hospitalized Children. Pediatrics. 1999:103:1050-1052.

5) American Academy of Pediatrics. Committee on Hospital Care. Family-Centered Care and the Pediatrician's Role. Pediatrics. 2003:112:691-696.

6) Kaushal R, et al. Medication errors and adverse drug events in pediatric inpatients. JAMA 2001;285:2114-2120.

7) American Academy of Pediatrics. Surgical Advisory Panel. Guidelines for referral to Pediatric Surgical Sub specialists. Pediatrics. 2002;110:187-191.

8) Gausche-Hill M, Schmitz C and Lewis RJ. Pediatric Preparedness of US Emergency Departments: A 2003 Survey. Pediatrics. 2007;120:1229-1237.

9) Institute of Medicine, Committee on Quality Health Care in America. *Crossing the Quality Chiasm: A New health System for the 21st Century.* Washington, DC. The National Academies Press;2001.

WEB SITES

American Academy of Pediatrics *www.aap.org*
Agency for Healthcare Quality Research *www.ahrq.gov*
The Joint Commission *www.jointcommission.org*
National Association of Children's Hospitals *www.chidlrenshospitals.net*

Psychiatric Treatments

Arnold Winston, M.D. and Michael Serby, M.D.

Patients need to have as much information as possible to make good decisions about their care. Knowing how to obtain this information, who to talk to and what to ask is generally a daunting and difficult task. Unfortunately, many patients find it difficult to formulate appropriate questions and even when they are able to do so have trouble pursuing these questions with their physicians. In this chapter we will discuss the questions that patients often ask us as well as those that often are not asked, and answer these questions in a clear, direct and down-to-earth manner. These issues are particularly important in psychiatry because of the stigma often associated with psychiatric illness. It is our hope that by directly confronting and answering these questions, psychiatry patients will have enough information and confidence in our field to seek necessary treatment without feeling stigmatized.

How do I know if I need counseling or psychiatric/psychological help?

There are many reasons to seek psychiatric care or counseling. A major reason is often the presence of uncomfortable and painful symptoms, such as anxiety, depression, sleeplessness, eating problems and difficulty functioning and managing the requirements of everyday life. In addition, many individuals will consider getting psychiatric help for interpersonal or relationship problems and difficulties at work or in school. For example, a man may have a problem developing a close relationship with a woman and over the course of a number of years does not enter into a stable and caring relationship.

Psychotherapy or counseling can help such an individual develop a satisfying and long-term relationship. Work or school problems can cause considerable suffering and poor performance, leading to diminished self-esteem and financial hardship.

These kinds of difficulties can result from interpersonal problems, depression, anxiety, as well as learning and attentional problems.

Some individuals may have more severe problems or symptoms, such as a loss of reality testing, identity problems, hyperactivity, disorganized thinking, and visions or voices. Others may have memory problems, confusion, disorientation, and other cognitive symptoms. Individuals with severe problems and safety concerns should be evaluated as quickly as possible and may need hospitalization.

What types of treatment or psychotherapy are available and how will I know which will be best for me?

There are many types of psychotherapy and varieties of different medications for psychiatric or mental health problems. The best way to find out what you need is to make an appointment for an evaluation with a mental health professional: a psychiatrist, psychologist or social worker. The evaluation should be in the form of an information gathering session to enable the doctor (therapist) to learn about your current problems, past problems, traumatic events in your life, your early life, your family and relationship experiences, school and work history and about any medical problems that you have or had in the past. After gathering this information, the doctor will be in a position to make a diagnosis and preliminary treatment plan and discuss recommendations with you about what type of treatment would be best for you. This would include the type of psychotherapy recommended and whether or not medication is indicated.

What kind of doctor will I need? Do I need a psychiatrist, psychologist or social worker to provide counseling or psychotherapy and are there different types of psychotherapy? What are the differences in these three specialties and what do they do?

Psychiatrists, psychologists, and social workers can all provide psychotherapy. However, there are many different types of psychotherapy and an individual therapist is unlikely to be an expert in more than one or two different psychotherapies. In general, all recognized therapies produce about the same results with just a few exceptions. These exceptions include individuals with anxiety disorders, including generalized anxiety disorder, post-traumatic stress disorder, panic disorder, and obsessive-compulsive disorder, which are best treated with cognitive-behavioral therapy.

Of the three types of professionals, only psychiatrists can prescribe medication. If you need medication at some point in your treatment you should see a psychiatrist. If you started treatment with a psychologist or social worker and need medication, you will need to see both a psychiatrist and nonpsychiatrist. Only a psychiatrist can provide both medication and psychotherapy.

Will I be informed about my diagnosis and what to expect about improvement or cure? What kind of goals can I have about improving or changing my life?

Your doctor should inform you about your diagnosis—explain its meaning—and answer any questions you have about your diagnosis. Your doctor should describe the available treatment approaches which might be best for you and the expected improvement for your problem or illness. You and your doctor should discuss the goals of treatment so that you have a clear understanding about what you can realistically accomplish. Goals can include a decrease or disappearance of symptoms, improvement in relationships with others and in work and school performance.

How often will I need to be seen and how long do typical sessions last? Does psychotherapy need to go on for years and years?

Most psychotherapy sessions are scheduled on a weekly basis, although some patients may be seen more frequently if necessary. It is generally best to schedule the same day and hour each week. Psychotherapy sessions generally last 45 to 50 minutes, although the initial evaluation session may require more time. Medication visits tend to run from 15 to 20 minutes. Psychotherapy does not need to go on for years and years. The length of treatment depends on such things as severity of illness, treatment goals and progress in treatment.

What can I expect to happen in a counseling or psychotherapy session?

What occurs in psychotherapy sessions depends on the type of psychotherapy that a patient receives. In dynamic exploratory psychotherapy, patients talk about their current problems, past problems and experiences with important people in their lives and the focus is on both feelings and thoughts. The therapist listens, asks questions, makes connections between past and current experiences, and at times explores the patient/therapist relationship. The emphasis is on an in-depth exploration and resolution of conflicts and problems. Supportive psychotherapy focuses on reducing symptoms, improving self-esteem, and helping patients to function in everyday life. The emphasis is on current functioning and not on an in-depth exploration of conflicts. In cognitive-behavioral therapy the therapist concentrates on problematic thinking and behavior, explores and helps correct dysfunctional thinking, uses stress reduction procedures and gives patients homework to do between sessions.

What about medications for psychiatric problems? Are they always necessary? Don't all medications produce side effects? Will I be giving up control of myself and my emotions if I take medication? If I take medication does that mean I'm weak and can't figure out how to deal with life's problems?

Medications are not always necessary. For some disorders, such as depression and anxiety, medication and psychotherapy may be equally effective. Patient preference can be an important determinant in deciding between medication and psychotherapy for these disorders. In some disorders, such as schizophrenia or bipolar disorder, medication is an absolute necessity, but psychotherapy can also be helpful for these disorders when combined with medication. Medications generally help to decrease symptoms and enable patients to feel more comfortable. Medications generally lead to an increase in the control and processing of difficult impulses and emotions as well as emotional stability, which can help an individual deal with stressful situations and life's problems.

How will I know when to stop treatment?

How long an individual needs to be in psychiatric treatment or psychotherapy depends on a number of factors. These include the severity of the problem, your goals for the treatment and how quickly you can meet your goals. How often you will need to be seen depends on the type of treatment you receive. If you are receiving medication you will generally be seen once a week for the first month or two, and then less frequently, perhaps every other week for the next month and then monthly. Individuals in psychotherapy are generally seen once or twice a week and stay on this type of schedule until therapy is completed.

What about electroconvulsive therapy? Is it safe? For which diagnoses is it useful? Can it be done on an outpatient basis?

Electroconvulsive therapy (ECT) is an unusually safe and effective treatment that is particularly useful for severe depression that does not respond to medication and psychotherapy. It produces remission of depression in 70% of people with severe depression. It may produce temporary confusion lasting approximately 30 minutes and some memory problems for events immediately surrounding the procedure. Memory function returns to normal quickly, allowing people to recall past events without a problem. It is administered in a hospital by a psychiatrist, assisted by an anesthesiologist and a nurse. ECT can be done for hospitalized patients and on an outpatient or ambulatory basis, with treatments administered three times a week for two to three weeks.

What about hospitalization? What are the benefits of hospitalization?

People may experience significant changes in their mood, thinking and functioning. If these changes are severe enough, a brief period in the hospital can be very helpful. Deep depression with insomnia, loss of appetite, weight loss, and particularly suicidal wishes is one indication for admission. Others include disorganized and confused thought, mental agitation and restlessness, extreme fear and anxiety, and disturbing visions or voices.

A hospital stay allows people to be treated for these conditions in a supportive environment, away from everyday pressures. The staff are experienced in devising a treatment plan specifically for each patient. Patients may benefit greatly from those approaches. The average stay is approximately two weeks. Patients are discharged back to the community after much consideration of their subsequent treatment needs.

What does inpatient treatment consist of?

Each patient is treated by a team of doctors, nurses, social workers and activity and occupational therapists. Patients meet with various staff members daily, individually and in groups. Therapy sessions focus on major problems and concerns. Activities are designed to foster relaxation and to help people focus on constructive and rewarding pursuits. Most patients will receive at least one medication. Commonly prescribed drugs include anti-depressants, tranquilizers, mood stabilizers and sleeping pills. The use of medications is thoroughly discussed with patients. Any co-existing medical problems, such as diabetes or hypertension, will be monitored and treated.

Families and friends are encouraged to visit and may discuss treatment in accordance with patients' wishes.

Patients also have access to a patient representative and to an independent Mental Hygiene Legal Service.

What are the other patients like?

Patients with multiple kinds of emotional and behavioral problems are admitted. An attempt is made to treat similar kinds of conditions on specialized units. There is a geriatric unit and a unit for patients with drug and alcohol problems. Frequently, people find comfort and understanding from their fellow patients.

At all times, the staff is quick to address any concerns patients have, including ones relating to other patients. The units are safe and therapeutic.

Is there student training in the inpatient units?

There are medical students, residents, and fellows, all of whom are training in Psychiatry at various levels. They are thoroughly supervised by licensed attending psychiatrists. There are also supervised trainees in Psychology, Nursing and Occupational Therapy. This academic atmosphere contributes to a high level of knowledge and clinical skills.

Conclusion

In summary, patients should feel free to ask questions of their psychiatrists and all staff involved in their care. A well-informed patient who understands the treatment process will be more comfortable and make better progress in resolving problems and reducing symptoms. In addition, in recent years psychiatry has been making great strides in understanding and identifying the underlying causes of psychiatric illness. This progress has helped to develop new medications and better and more varied psychotherapies. There is every reason to believe that this progress will continue resulting in our ability to provide better and better treatments for our patients

Dealing With Problems
in the Hospital

What If I Am Concerned About My Care in the Hospital?

Joann Coffin, RHIA, CPHQ and
David Bernard, MD, FRCP, FACP

It is very important that as a patient in the hospital, you are fully informed about all aspects of your care and that you feel confident you are receiving safe and high quality care. A number of avenues are available for you to take if you need reassurance on these matters. Members of the hospital staff are responsible for answering your questions. For example, physicians are expected to take time to explain the reasons for the tests you are having, the treatment you are receiving and the basic cause of your problem. They should also be available to you to answer any questions you may have. Listed below are some examples of situations that may arise during your hospital stay and the best way for you to resolve them.

Who should I speak to if something is not going well in the hospital?

If you feel something is not going well with your treatment, or you have a concern about your care, it is very important that you share this information with your nurse or your doctor. If you are not comfortable addressing the issue with one of your care givers, you may call the *Patient Representative Department*. (Most hospitals have a Patient Representative Department, but if they do not then you should call the Administration of the hospital). Patient representatives can help you understand hospital policies and procedures and answer any questions you may have about patients' rights. They can also assist in getting information for you and facilitate communication with other hospital staff. Patient representatives work on behalf of patients in order to help them and their families resolve issues and obtain information and/or services.

What should I do if the issue does not seem to be resolved?

If your issues are not resolved by your doctor, nurse, or the patient representative, you may directly call any of the members of the hospital's most senior leaders. These include the Chief Operating Officer, the Chief Nursing Officer, the Chief Medical Officer or even the Chief Executive Officer. If you are not comfortable speaking with a member of the hospital staff, you may voice your concerns directly to one of two organizations who oversee, license or monitor the hospital's compliance with regulatory issues. They are The Joint Commission, at 800-994-6610, or the local State Department of Health (DOH). The Joint Commission is a National Accrediting body whose mission is to improve the quality and safety of patient care. Most hospitals are surveyed regularly by The Joint Commission.

How quickly should I expect that someone will get back to me?

An initial acknowledgement of your request for information or resolution of a concern should be received within 24 hours. It may take longer to fully investigate and respond to the issue.

If I see something that concerns me, should I say something and risk the staff taking it out on me?

You should absolutely always report anything that concerns you. Hospitals expect and welcome being told about issues of concern to patients. This is one of the most important sources of information that hospitals use to enable them to constantly improve the way they operate. You should never feel you will be discriminated against if you report a concern. If you are not comfortable sharing your concerns with the staff immediately caring for you, you may speak to a Patient Representative or to any other hospital staff person, including the senior leaders mentioned before or one of the Directors of Nursing.

What if the hospital does not take my concerns seriously, what can I do?

If the hospital does not take your concerns seriously, you may call the regulatory organizations mentioned before, namely The Joint Commission or the State Department of Health. The Joint Commission has published a brochure called "The Speak-up Brochure" which is generally included in the package of information given to patients on admission to hospital. The brochure encourages patients to become involved with their care and explains how to do so. It is available in several languages. New York State has also published a booklet entitled "Your Rights as a Hospital Patient in NYS". This booklet contains information on how to refer issues and concerns to the Department of Health directly.

What should I do if I am told that I cannot reach my doctor because it's a night or a weekend?

A doctor is available to speak to you any time of the day or night, any day of the week—a 24/7 commitment. It may not always be your own doctor, since another doctor may be covering your care, but it will always be a doctor with access to your medical information and the treatment you are receiving. If your nurse is unable to contact your doctor for you, just ask to see the Nursing Supervisor on call. The Nursing Supervisor is a senior nurse who is in the hospital at all times and available to speak to you at any time about any, concerns and will help to contact your physician.

Are There Ways I Can Contribute To Make My Care Safe?

There are indeed specific ways in which you can help make your hospital stay safe. Many of these are included in "The Joint Commission Speak-up Brochure" included in the package which is given to patients at the time of admission at many hospitals. For example, following certain practices to prevent infection can have a positive impact on your hospital experience. Key examples include the following:

- As outlined above, keep your health care team informed of issues, concerns, and symptoms.
- To prevent infections please remember not to share your belongings with other patients and to wash your hands as often as necessary. It is important to discourage family members and friends who are sick from visiting you. Make sure your identity band (ID band) is checked before receiving medications.

Are Specific Resources That Deal With some Of These Issues Available For Patients?

Indeed they are. When you are admitted to hospital, you will be given an "admission package". This should contain several useful resources that expand on the issues discussed above. They include:

a. Literature from the local Department of Health, which includes information on "Your Rights As a Patient in New York State"

b. The Joint Commission Speak-Up Brochure
c. A Patient Guide Book. This includes information on:

- The Joint Commission
- The Department of Health
- The roles of the Patient Representative and how to contact them
- The Hospital Ethics Committee and its role
- The Department of Social Work and how they can help you
- Hospital Services
- Safety Information
- Discharge Information
- An Important Message from "Medicare
- Privacy Practices

Rapid Response Teams

Sam Acqah, M.D.

Modern hospital systems have slowly added to the traditional patient care goals of disease diagnosis and treatment by developing multiple systems to improve both the quality and safety of patient care. One of the measures advocated by the Institute of Healthcare Improvement (1) to improve patient safety by preventing unnecessary deaths is the institution of "rapid response" systems. These systems were designed with the intent of providing prompt and effective attention to any patient who is recognized by a family member, visitor, or employee of the hospital to be at risk of deterioration or who suffers a deterioration of any severity from any cause. This newfound emphasis on prevention of clinical deterioration is in marked contrast to systems traditionally designed to only respond to limited types of emergencies such as cardiac arrests and with the responses designed solely for *after* such arrests occur. Focusing on prevention reveals a lot about the evolution of quality and safety in a health care system.

Having worked as a critical care physician for over ten years, predominantly in the era before rapid response teams became commonplace, I have been a firsthand witness to its benefits in improving patient care. Many clinicians were initially apprehensive of the new system, largely due to the presumed effects of added responsibilities to an already stressful schedule. However, over time the rewards of seeing fewer emergencies in hospital patients as well as the development of a rapid and efficient system of transferring critically ill patients to units where the level of care could more closely match the severity of illness has definitively won over the majority of intensive care physicians.

Traditionally, if a patient was noted to require urgent medical attention or a higher level of attention, the process of achieving this goal was quite laborious for hospital employees and clinicians. For example, a nurse would first try to find the "covering" doctor who was not always physically present on each ward.

The doctor would then have to be paged, and although they would attempt to respond as quickly as possible, they often were not the most experienced or most skilled in the diagnosis and treatment of critically ill patients. Such a doctor would then have to call for more experienced or specialized help, again inviting more delays in the provision of potentially life-saving medical treatment.

Rapid response teams were designed to circumvent all such barriers and delays to prompt medical intervention. Once the need for such care is recognized, a simple telephone activation of a "Rapid Response" team is all that is needed for highly skilled and experienced clinicians to appear at the patient's bedside with the necessary equipment for emergency medical conditions.

What is an RRT? Is there national data to suggest they are effective?

Rapid Response Teams are specialized teams created by hospitals to take care of patients who develop a rapidly deteriorating clinical condition on a standard hospital ward. Although such hospital wards are well-designed to provide routine medical care for the majority of medical conditions encountered in a hospital, they are ill-suited for the care of a severely ill or rapidly deteriorating patient. The RRT team is a way to bring critical care expertise, resources and equipment to a patient's bedside to help prevent further deterioration. Such a team has two main goals: the immediate stabilization of the patient, and the rapid transfer to an intensive care unit, if deemed necessary.

A rapid response team is a multidisciplinary team staffed by various combinations of health care employees, most commonly by one or more of the following: Critical care physician, nursing supervisor, respiratory therapist, registered nurse and transport employees. Such teams are known by a variety of different names such as Rapid Response Teams, Emergency Medical Teams and Critical Care Outreach Teams. Research data has shown that the institution of Rapid Response Teams result in fewer numbers of cardiac arrest calls on hospital wards, decreased length of hospital and ICU stays and a decrease in the number of emergency ICU admissions. More recent data suggest that such teams may in fact decrease the risk of dying while in a hospital. (2)

What should a staff member do to call a RRT?

Any and all hospital employees or visitors are empowered to activate a Rapid Response Team, from bedside nurses and physicians to family members, from housekeeping staff to security guards, too. The success of the Rapid Response Team is dependant on the ability of personnel who work closely with the patient and first witness or suspect deterioration to immediately call an RRT so as to avoid delay in treatment. "Calling an RRT" is as simple as picking up the nearest telephone. To activate an RRT team, you commonly call the hospital operator by dialing 0 or the emergency line, which varies by hospital but can often be found on the telephone or by asking any nearby employee. If the situation ever arises whereby the RRT response is thought inadequate either in response time or adequacy to the clinical condition (such as a cardiac arrest), then a Cardiac Arrest Code can be called, with the number again varying by hospital although any hospital operator can activate such a team as well. Once any emergency team is activated, the caller should then listen for the public address announcement to be made and then stay by the patient's side until the team arrives.

Can I or my family member call an RRT?

Yes. If at any time a family member feels there has been a serious change in a patient's condition and help is either not immediately available or is delayed for any reason, they can call an RRT by immediately dialing the emergency line, if known, or the hospital operator at 0. The operator will answer the phone and the family member must then state that they are calling a RRT and promptly provide the patient's name and location.

What is the difference between an RRT and a Code?

Rapid Response Teams are designed to respond to immediately assess any worrisome change in a patient's condition with the aim of preventing the patient from deteriorating to a cardiac arrest. The purpose of the RRT team is to immediately stabilize such a patient and then rapidly transfer the patient to an intensive care unit where they can receive closer monitoring or more aggressive interventions as needed so as to avoid a cardiac arrest. A "code" is called any time a patient stops breathing or their heart stops beating. In this situation, a more specialized "code" team is activated to respond to this situation. Although most hospitals design and staff these teams as separate entities, in practice, RRT teams are as capable of treating cardiac arrest patients as the traditional "code" teams.

References

1. Institute of Health Care Improvement (*www.ihi.org*)
2. Rapid response systems: A systematic review. Winters Bradford, Phd,MD, Julius Cuong MD, Pronovost, Peter PhD MD CCM May 2007

Pain in the Hospital

Russell Portenoy, M.D.

Will I always experience pain when I go into the hospital?

No one can predict whether a patient will experience pain, but it is obvious that the potential exists for many patients admitted to a hospital. Patients admitted for surgery expect to experience some pain, of course, but it is equally likely that other types of problems will create the potential for pain. These include admissions after trauma such as automobile accidents; admissions for illnesses that are associated with a high likelihood of pain, such as cancer or HIV disease; admissions that lead to a prolonged period of bed rest; and admissions for any reason that happen to people who have a history of chronic pain such as low back pain, arthritis or headaches.

During the past three decades, the problem of pain in the hospital has been the object of many scientific studies. These studies have yielded important conclusions, including the following:

- Pain is very common in hospitals, but uncontrolled pain—pain that is distressing to the patient and family, pain that interferes with sleep and the ability to function in the hospital, pain that slows down discharge from the hospital—is the real issue. Simply put, uncontrolled pain is bad for a person's health and well-being. Hospitals must take specific actions to minimize the occurrence of uncontrolled pain, whatever its cause.
- Historically, physicians and nurses have not done a good enough job in assessing patients for pain and reacting to it when it occurs. This observation led a major professional society—the American Pain Society—to propose guidelines for pain management in the hospital, the most important part of which was: **Make pain visible by asking about it and documenting where the doctors and nurses can see**

it. Reacting to this guideline, the national accrediting organization for hospitals, The Joint Commission, created standards for quality pain care a few years ago. These standards were based on making pain visible and promoted the concept of pain as the "5th Vital Sign." This means that hospital staff should be evaluating patients for their pain just as intensively as they monitor other vital signs, like pulse, blood pressure and temperature.

- Patients often under-report pain and they do so for a variety of reasons. They may not want to be seen as "complainers," or to distract the physician from efforts to treat the disease. They may believe that poorly controlled pain is "normal" for the problem that brought them to the hospital, or that there is nothing that can be done. They may fear pain treatment, like opioid (so-called narcotic) medications. All these perceptions are problems or are inaccurate. Patients must not be shy about reporting pain. Good hospitals want patients to be a "partner" in the treatment of pain. This means being open and honest, and if necessary, even a bit "pushy"—to make sure that this problem is dealt with by the professionals caring for the patient.

How do I know if my pain could be better controlled?

Pain is usually not eliminated. The goal of pain treatment should be to reduce the intensity of pain to a level that is tolerable and allows sleep and improving function, and to do so without the experience of severe side effects from medicines or other therapies. Although it is true that not all pains can be effectively managed, even with state-of-the-art therapy, the reality is that the vast majority of pain problems in the hospital can be satisfactorily treated. Patients who are experiencing pain that is, even periodically, above a tolerable level, or pain that is interfering with sleep or function, should report this to the nurses and physicians. Treatment should usually be changed in an effort to improve it. There should be an open dialogue about pain between patients and staff, and in the unusual event that pain cannot be better controlled, the patient should understand the reasons for this and any options for a future plan of care.

How should the hospital staff be assessing my pain level?

Although pain specialists emphasize that pain "assessment," which includes information about the location, quality, timing, impact and other features of the pain, is not the same as "measurement" of pain severity, it is now well accepted that pain assessment can begin with a question about severity. In the hospital, the concept of pain as the "5th Vital Sign" typically means that the staff should inquire about the presence of pain and its severity on a regular basis. After surgery, this might be every few hours, and in other settings, it could be twice a day.

If a patient says that he or she is experiencing pain, the severity measurement typically uses either a verbal scale or a so-called numeric scale. A verbal rating scale measures pain using descriptive words, such as *none, mild, moderate* and *severe*. A numeric scale usually involves this question: "On a scale from zero to ten, where zero is no pain and ten is the worst pain imaginable, how would you rate your pain right now?" Occasionally, other scales are used to accomplish this measurement. The important point is that the patient should be asked about the presence and severity of pain on a regular basis, that the same scale should be used repeatedly, that the scale that is used should be in a language understood by the patient, and the results from this measurement should be recorded where the doctors and nurses can see it.

How do I know if I can ask for more pain medication?

In the hospital, most patients with pain severe enough to need treatment are treated with medication. The medications that are used for pain include acetaminophen, anti-inflammatory drugs such as ibuprofen, and the opioids such as morphine. Opioids typically are selected when the pain is severe, such as after surgery or trauma, or in the setting of some illnesses, such as cancer, sickle cell anemia and many others. In every case, the doctor should take into account the medical condition of the patient when selecting a drug for pain and choosing an initial dose.

The way that patients respond to all the pain-relieving drugs may differ greatly. Sometimes the drug and initial dose is just right, and pain control is prompt and reliable. Sometimes a reasonable selection results in poor control of pain or the experience of side effects like nausea or sleepiness. In every case, the therapy should be monitored by the nurses and physicians, and in every case, patients should not hesitate to report the way that they feel—either to describe improvement, or to report that pain continues to be poorly controlled or a new symptom is occurring. Patients should never hesitate to ask for more pain medication if pain is poorly controlled, or at least to say that more help is needed. The doctor may or may not decide that the best course of action is to increase the dose—there may be other things that are more likely to work, or safer—but there is no way for the doctor to know that a change is needed unless the patient reports it.

Should I be concerned about an overdose from pain medications?

Many patients or family members express concern about pain medications, specifically the opioid drugs (also known as the narcotics). These concerns sometimes revolve around the fear of addiction and sometimes focus on the risk of overdose or side effects. Doctors and nurses should openly discuss these concerns with patients. The following are the key points: 1) Addiction is a disease characterized by intense craving for a drug and use of the drug for its psychic effects. Drug abuse is using an illegal drug or a prescribed drug in a manner not prescribed. If a person without a known drug addiction uses a pain medication, particularly in the hospital, the risk that addiction can develop is believed to be almost zero. If a person has an addiction and needs pain medication in the hospital, the risk that the addiction will be made worse by the pain medication is similarly miniscule. If a person is prescribed pain medication in the hospital, doctors and nurses expect that there will be no abuse problems. Even if a person abuses drugs outside the hospital, pain is typically treated with whatever medication is needed, and treatment should proceed without problems as long as the patient acts responsibly and there is good communication between the hospital staff and the patient.

Side effects are common with pain medication and include: sleepiness or mental clouding, nausea, itch and constipation. The patient should tell the doctors and nurses if these symptoms are distressing, and treatments can be changed in an effort to reduce them. Serious side effects and overdose are extremely rare in a hospital environment. As long as they are appropriately prescribed, opioid medications are considered to be quite safe for patients.

How do I know if a PCA pump is right for me?

PCA—patient-controlled analgesia—is the concept that pain control is likely to be better if a patient is given the opportunity to adjust his or her pain medication. Devices known as PCA pumps have been developed so that patients can push a button and deliver small amounts of medication, usually intravenously, as often as they need it. The pump can be programmed to prevent the delivery of too much medication. The PCA approach has been around for about 30 years and usually is preferred for the management of acute pain in the hospital, and sometimes for the management of chronic pain as well. Doctors or nurses usually suggest the use of a PCA pump very routinely for some types of pain problems. When it is suggested, patients should ask questions or raise concerns, so that they can learn the reasons that it may have advantages and get reassured that the approach is safe.

When do I need a consult from a pain specialist?

Pain medicine is a subspecialty. This means that physicians who are interested in this field take extra training and can become Board Certified in pain management. Other professionals, including nurses, can also obtain advanced training in pain management. Hospitals that provide excellent pain care typically have pain specialists available to help patients who have pain that is difficult to control or requires special techniques. The most sophisticated hospitals offer several types of pain consultations: 1) an Acute Pain Service, which may include nurses or physicians and is available to help the surgeons and others deal with acute postoperative pain (such as PCA pumps); 2) a Pain Consultation Service, which may include physicians and other specialists and is available to help in the care of any patients with difficult-to-control pain; and 3) an ambulatory (outpatient) pain practice, which typically includes a team of specialists and can receive referrals of patients who are discharged from the hospital and will continue to need help in the management of pain. Patients should know that these specialists exist and are available to consult if needed. Patients whose pain remains poorly controlled despite the efforts of their physicians, or who are experiencing side effects or other problems from pain treatment, or who have a pain problem that has proved difficult to diagnose should discuss the possibility of a consultation by a pain specialist, in the hospital or after discharge.

References or Resources for Pain

www.StopPain.org—website for the Department of Pain Medicine and Palliative Care at Beth Israel Medical Center.

www.painfoundation.org—website for the American Pain Foundation, which has extensive information about pain management for patients.

Language and Communication Issues

Susan Gold, MSW

What should I do if I am not comfortable speaking English in the hospital?

In many states, the law requires all hospitals to provide interpreter services, free of charge. If you are uncomfortable speaking English, you should ask for an interpreter in the language of your choice. If at any time this is not offered, you should request it. It is your right.

Is it okay to have a family member translate for me?

It is the hospital's responsibility to provide you with free interpreter services. However, if you prefer to use a friend, family member or significant other, you can choose to do so.

If I am deaf what type of help in the hospital can I expect?

In many states, hospitals are required to provide Sign Language interpreter services to all deaf patients. This can be provided through the use of on-site interpreters, TTY telephone services as well as electronic (video) system—all of which provide translation to the hearing impaired. These services should be provided throughout the entire course of your medical care. If at any time interpreter services are not offered, you should request them. It is your right.

What should I do if I cannot read and I am asked to sign a form in the hospital?

If you are unable to read, you should ask that the form be read aloud to you in the language in which you are most comfortable. If it is not English, you should ask the hospital to provide you with a translator.

If I don't understand what my doctor is talking about when he/she explains something to me, what should I do?

Understanding your medical condition can often be complicated and overwhelming. If you do not understand what the doctor or any other health care professional is telling you, you should always feel free to ask them to explain it to you again. Sometimes it is helpful if the doctor writes down or draws diagrams describing the key components of your medical condition. It is often helpful to have a friend, family member or significant other with you when speaking with your doctor. It may also be helpful to ask the doctor if you can explain back to him/her what you understand to be your medical condition.

Who can I speak to if I have questions about the availability of language services?

Most hospitals are required to have a Language Access Coordinator who is available to assist you with any question you may have. In addition, many hospitals have a Patient Representative Department which can help guide you.

Protecting Your Rights and Beliefs in the Hospital

Robert Schiller, M.D.

Is there such a thing as a Patients Bill of Rights?

Most states have laws protecting patient's rights that also comply with federal guidelines. For example, if you are treated in New York State, you are protected by New York State law which has a Patients Bill of Rights. A copy of this Bill of Rights is at the end of this section. Briefly these rights include:

- access to language translators if necessary
- no discrimination in treatment by race, color, religion, sex, national origin, sexual orientation or ability to pay
- receive care in a clean setting that is respectful and safe
- know the name of the doctor who is in charge of your care
- know the names of all the doctors and nurses caring for you
- have complete information about the diagnosis and treatment of your medical condition
- have all the information you need in a way that you understand to give consent to any test or procedure
- be able to decline any test or treatment or participate in any research
- trust that the privacy of your health information will not be violated
- be able to complain about your treatment without fear of being mistreated
- be able to review and understand your medical record

There is no federal law, so this applies only to New York State. There are federal guidelines, and a copy of this is also attached. However, there are some patient rights that apply only to patients who have Medicare and/or Medicaid, and certain managed care plans.

Should I ask my doctor about an advanced directive if I don't have one?

Yes, you should ask your doctor about advance directives and you should know that under New York State law, all doctors are required to inform patients and their families about the need for an advanced directive. An Advance Directive means that you have identified someone (called a health care proxy) who would make medical decisions for you, should you be unable to make them yourself. This person can be a spouse, a child, any relative or close friend. It cannot be your doctor. It is very important that this person clearly understand your preferences for medical treatment, especially regarding end of life care, and the use of artificial nutrition and hydration.

What if I don't want anyone else to have information about my medical condition, including my friends and family?

The laws in New York State regarding patient privacy are very clear. You are the only person who can decide if anyone else should know about your medical condition, including family. When you are admitted to the hospital you should have information on how the hospital protects the privacy of health information. If you have any concerns about who should know about your personal health information including drug or alcohol use, HIV status, or any test results, you should tell your doctors and your nurses as soon as possible. You should tell them the specific people who should have this information and who should not. They are required to follow your wishes.

You also have the right to review and have a copy of your complete medical record, and you have the right to request additions to the record if you feel it is not complete or accurate.

What should I do if I hear that information is being given out about me without my permission?

You should ask to speak with someone from the hospital administration, usually this is someone from the patient representative department. When you are admitted, the hospital provides you with information on what to do if you feel your privacy has been violated.

What if I would rather have my spouse or children make my decisions for me?

You have the right to have anyone you wish to help make your medical decisions for you, including your spouse or child. It is preferable that you identify one person as the main decision maker and choose another as an alternative if the first person is unavailable. This is very helpful to your doctors and nurses. Also it is advisable to discuss this as a family prior to any serious medical decisions, so all family members understand your wishes and can honor them. Finally, the primary and secondary decision makers should be documented in a health care proxy form that you need to sign. Please keep the original and have a copy for the hospital staff when you get admitted.

I have special religious beliefs; will these be respected in the hospital (e.g. Jehovah's Witness)?

By law in New York State you must receive medical treatment that does not discriminate against you based upon your religious beliefs. If you are aware of any religious beliefs or practices that would influence your medical treatment or hospital stay, you are advised to identify them even before you go to the hospital and let your family members know. This would include the use of blood products such as transfusions or certain dietary preferences. If you feel your religious beliefs have been violated, you are encouraged to contact the Hospital administration and have your concerns addressed, and file a complaint if necessary.

If I disagree with the way my doctors are wanting to care for me or my family, is there a way to get some additional advice on the issue?

You have the right to the best possible care. If you disagree or have questions regarding your treatment, you can ask for another doctor to evaluate your condition. Usually you can contact the patient representative department for help with this.

What should I do if the doctors ask for a family meeting or an Ethics consult regarding me or my family member?

If your doctors are requesting a family meeting, it is likely that there is a complex or difficult decision regarding your treatment or discharge plans from the hospital. It is very helpful to have key family members participate in this discussion. You should decide who should be present and who makes the final decision.

An ethics consult is usually requested by the doctors or nurses caring for you when they have a difficult decision regarding your treatment that usually involves potentially life threatening or life altering medical decisions.

Is there someone that can serve as a Patient Advocate if I have no one else to look after me?

Yes, most hospitals have a Patient Representative Department, and you can ask them. Also, you can ask your doctor, nurse or social worker, as well as any clergy or religious leader from your community for help in identifying a patient advocate.

New York State Patients' Bill of Rights

If you are not receiving care in New York, ask the hospital administration for a copy of your state's Bill or Rights. In New York, as a patient in a hospital, you have the right, consistent with law, to:

(1) Understand and use these rights. If for any reason you do not understand or you need help, the hospital MUST provide assistance, including an interpreter.
(2) Receive treatment without discrimination as to race, color, religion, sex, national origin, disability, sexual orientation or source of payment.
(3) Receive considerate and respectful care in a clean and safe environment free of unnecessary restraints.
(4) Receive emergency care if you need it.
(5) Be informed of the name and position of the doctor who will be in charge of your care in the hospital.
(6) Know the names, positions and functions of any hospital staff involved in your care and refuse their treatment, examination or observation.
(7) A no smoking room.
(8) Receive complete information about your diagnosis, treatment and prognosis.
(9) Receive all the information that you need to give informed consent for any proposed procedure or treatment. This information shall include the possible risks and benefits of the procedure or treatment.
(10) Receive all the information you need to give informed consent for an order not to resuscitate. You also have the right to designate an individual to give this consent for you if you are too ill to do so. If you would like additional information, please ask for a copy of the pamphlet "Do Not Resuscitate Orders—A Guide for Patients and Families."
(11) Refuse treatment and be told what effect this may have on your health.
(12) Refuse to take part in research. In deciding whether or not to participate, you have the right to a full explanation.

(13) Privacy while in the hospital and confidentiality of all information and records regarding your care.

(14) Participate in all decisions about your treatment and discharge from the hospital. The hospital must provide you with a written discharge plan and written description of how you can appeal your discharge.

(15) Review your medical record without charge. Obtain a copy of your medical record for which the hospital can charge a reasonable fee. You cannot be denied a copy solely because you cannot afford to pay.

(16) Receive an itemized bill and explanation of all charges.

(17) Complain without fear of reprisals about the care and services you are receiving and to have the hospital respond to you and if you request it, a written response. If you are not satisfied with the hospital's response, you can complain to the New York State Health Department. The hospital must provide you with the State Health Department telephone number.

(18) Authorize those family members and other adults who will be given priority to visit consistent with your ability to receive visitors.

(19) Make known your wishes in regard to anatomical gifts. You may document your wishes in your health care proxy or on a donor card, available from the hospital. Public Health Law(PHL)2803 (1)(g)Patient's Rights, 10NYCRR, 405.7,405.7(a)(1),405.7(c)

Web site:

http://www.health.state.ny.us/professionals/patients/patient_rights/docs/english.pdf

THE PATIENTS' BILL OF RIGHTS IN MEDICARE AND MEDICAID

Overview: On March 26, 1997, President Clinton created the Advisory Commission on Consumer Protection and Quality in the Health Care Industry and charged it with recommend[ing] such measures as may be necessary to promote and assure health care quality and value and protect consumers and workers in the health care system." As part of that charge, the President asked the Commission to develop a "Patients' Bill of Rights" in health care.

In February 1998, President Clinton directed the Department of Health and Human Services (HHS), along with the departments of Labor, Defense, and Veterans' Affairs and the Office of Personnel Management, to use their regulatory and administrative authority to bring their health programs into compliance with the Bill of Rights and Responsibilities.

HHS' Health Care Financing Administration (HCFA) has begun the work to establish new requirements for managed care plans participating in the Medicare program. It is also working to strengthen protections for beneficiaries enrolled in Medicaid managed care. In November 1998, HHS issued a report to the Vice President showing that it is moving aggressively to strengthen existing patient protections under Medicare and Medicaid.

When these regulations are fully implemented, Medicare and Medicaid will have among the strongest patients' protections in the country. The proposed regulations give HHS a variety of monitoring and enforcement tools, including suspension of payments, civil monetary penalties, and termination from the Medicare and Medicaid programs.

BACKGROUND: THE PRESIDENT'S ADVISORY COMMISSION ON CONSUMER PROTECTION AND QUALITY IN THE HEALTH CARE INDUSTRY AND THE PATIENTS' BILL OF RIGHTS

In November 1997, President Clinton's Advisory Commission on Consumer Protection and Quality on the Health Care Industry, in an Interim Report, issued the Patients' Bill of Rights and Responsibilities. The Commission's Final Report, "Quality First: Better Health Care for All Americans," was issued in March 1998.

Co-Chaired by Secretary of Health and Human Services Donna E. Shalala and Secretary of Labor Alexis M. Herman, the Commission had 34 members, including broad-based representation from consumers, businesses, labor, health care providers, health plans, and health care quality and financing experts.

The Patients' Bill of Rights and Responsibilities has three goals: to strengthen consumer confidence that the health care system is fair and responsive to consumer needs; to reaffirm the importance of a strong relationship between patients and their health care providers; and to reaffirm the critical role consumers play in safeguarding their own health. The Commission articulated seven sets of rights and one set of responsibilities:

- **The Right to Information.** Patients have the right to receive accurate, easily understood information to assist them in making informed decisions about their health plans, facilities and professionals.
- **The Right to Choose.** Patients have the right to a choice of health care providers that is sufficient to assure access to appropriate high-quality health care including giving women access to qualified specialists such as obstetrician-gynecologists and giving patients with serious medical conditions and chronic illnesses access to specialists.
- **Access to Emergency Services.** Patients have the right to access emergency health services when and where the need arises. Health plans should provide payment when a patient presents himself/herself to any emergency department with acute symptoms of sufficient severity "including severe pain" that a "prudent layperson" could reasonably expect the absence of medical attention to result in placing that consumer's health in serious jeopardy, serious impairment to bodily functions, or serious dysfunction of any bodily organ or part.
- **Being a Full Partner in Health Care Decisions.** Patients have the right to fully participate in all decisions related to their health care. Consumers who are unable to fully participate in treatment decisions have the right to be represented by parents, guardians, family members, or other conservators. Additionally, provider contracts should not contain any so-called "gag clauses" that restrict health professionals' ability to discuss and advise patients on medically necessary treatment options.
- **Care Without Discrimination.** Patients have the right to considerate, respectful care from all members of the health care industry at all times

and under all circumstances. Patients must not be discriminated against in the marketing or enrollment or in the provision of health care services, consistent with the benefits covered in their policy and/or as required by law, based on race, ethnicity, national origin, religion, sex, age, current or anticipated mental or physical disability, sexual orientation, genetic information, or source of payment.

- **The Right to Privacy.** Patients have the right to communicate with health care providers in confidence and to have the confidentiality of their individually-identifiable health care information protected. Patients also have the right to review and copy their own medical records and request amendments to their records.
- **The Right to Speedy Complaint Resolution.** Patients have the right to a fair and efficient process for resolving differences with their health plans, health care providers, and the institutions that serve them, including a rigorous system of internal review and an independent system of external review.
- **Taking on New Responsibilities.** In a health care system that affords patients rights and protections, patients must also take greater responsibility for maintaining good health.

MEDICARE AND MEDICAID COMPLIANCE WITH THE PATIENTS' BILL OF RIGHTS

While many of the protections articulated in the Bill of Rights are most relevant to individuals in managed care, such as those related to choice of providers and access to specialists, other protections such as complaints and appeals apply to beneficiaries not enrolled in managed care.

Medicare covers nearly 40 million individuals, of whom approximately 6.5 million, or 17 percent are currently enrolled in managed care arrangements. Medicaid covers an estimated 40 million people, of whom about half are in a managed care arrangement for some or all of their health care at some point during a year.

HHS has moved aggressively to strengthen existing patient protections under Medicare and Medicaid. On June 26, 1998, the Health Care Financing Administration (HCFA) published an Interim Final rule establishing new requirements for managed care arrangements participating in Medicare. On September 29, 1998, HCFA published a Notice of Proposed Rulemaking (NPRM) strengthening protections for Medicaid beneficiaries enrolled in managed care arrangements. Generally, the Medicare protections became effective on or before January 1, 1999, and were to be fully implemented by no later than December 31, 1999. States were required to implement all new protections within one year from the effective date of the final regulation for Medicaid, which was expected to be issued by mid-1999.

With the implementation of these regulations, Medicare and Medicaid has among the strongest patients' protections in the country. Specifically, HHS has been able to come into compliance for managed care enrollees with critical patient protections such as information disclosure, access to emergency services, patient participation in treatment decisions, and complaints and appeals. These regulations also expand patients' ability to choose their health care providers and to have ready access to specialists.

In a few areas, however, both Medicare and Medicaid currently lack the statutory authority to achieve full compliance with the Patients' Bill of Rights. For example, current legislative authority also does not permit full implementation of the right to medical record confidentiality. HHS has, however, separately submitted a report to the Congress laying out the parameters for federal legislation to protect the confidentiality of health records. Additionally, while Medicare and Medicaid managed care enrollees are currently protected to the full extent of the Patients' Bill of Rights with regard to respect and non-discrimination, the rules that prohibit discrimination under fee-for-service address some, but not all, categories of protection and providers included in the right as recommended by the Commission.

The regulations give HHS a variety of monitoring and enforcement tools including suspension of payments, civil money penalties, and termination from the Medicare and Medicaid programs. HHS will take all necessary actions to enforce the protections included in the Medicare and Medicaid regulations.

Specific Rights

Information Disclosure. Medicare and Medicaid require plans to provide critical information to consumers, both annually and upon request, that can enable them to make more informed choices about their health plans. Medicare's web site, www.medicare.gov, offers the "Medicare Compare" database to help beneficiaries evaluate different plans and decide which options are best, including comparative information about the quality of care provided to patients and about the level of satisfaction among patients with the care that they receive.

Choice of Providers and Plans. Regulations assure provider network adequacy, by requiring that medically necessary services be available 24 hours a day, 7 days a week to enrollees. Participating plans are required to offer women access to qualified women's health specialists for routine preventive care, and provide consumers with complex or serious medical conditions an adequate number of direct access visits to specialists under a plan of treatment. As has been the case since the start of these programs, Medicare and Medicaid beneficiaries who obtain their care on a fee-for-service basis can choose any provider who agrees to participate in these programs.

Access to Emergency Services. Emergency services will be covered when and where the need arises, in exact compliance with the Patients' Bill of Rights. Plans are not permitted to require preauthorization in order for an enrollee to obtain emergency services. In addition, the regulations articulate a standard for post-stabilization services that is applicable to both Medicare and Medicaid managed care enrollees. This policy identifies the obligation of the plan to pay for care provided after an emergency situation is stabilized, particularly when the plan fails to authorize such care on a timely basis.

Participation in Treatment Decisions. The regulations reflect existing and new policies that are consistent with this right, including information about treatment options and advance directives, physicians' financial disclosure and prohibition against "gag rules." Health plans are required to provide patients with easily understood information and the opportunity to decide among all treatment options—including no treatment—consistent with the informed consent process. Managed care organizations and providers are required to discuss the use of advance directives, or "living wills" with patients and their families and to abide by the wishes as expressed in an advanced directive, except where state law permits a provider to conscientiously object. Physicians are required to disclose to Medicare and Medicaid any financial arrangements that create incentives for limiting care. Plans are prohibited from penalizing or otherwise restricting the ability of health care providers to communicate with and advise Medicare and Medicaid patients about medically-necessary treatment options.

Respect and Nondiscrimination. Managed care enrollees are protected to the full extent of this right as articulated in the Bill of Rights, with regard to services, marketing and enrollment. Under fee-for-service, however, Medicare and Medicaid protections against discrimination are largely a function of federal anti-discrimination rules that apply to recipients of federal funds. These rules address some, but not all, categories of protection and providers included in the Bill of Rights. As a result, the fee-for-service aspects of Medicare and Medicaid are in only partial compliance with this right.

Confidentiality of Health Information. Plans are required to safeguard the privacy of any information that identifies a particular enrollee by ensuring that information from the plan (or copies of records) be released only to authorized individuals, that unauthorized individuals cannot gain access to or alter patient records, and that original medical records must be released only in accordance with federal or state law, court orders or subpoenas. In Medicaid, plans are required to establish procedures to address the confidentiality and privacy of minors, subject to applicable federal and state law.

While current federal laws and related regulations protect certain written records from disclosure outside of Medicare and Medicaid, such protections do not extend to all written records, nor to verbal communications between enrollees and providers. Protection of communication between patients and providers is a matter of state law, many of which do not afford the protections included in this right. Moreover, not all providers under Medicare and Medicaid are subject to federal laws on privacy. The Secretary's Privacy Recommendations to Congress (September 1997), when enacted, brought all beneficiary information obtained by Medicare and Medicaid providers and plans, as well as the programs and their contractors, into compliance with this right as articulated in the Bill of Rights.

Complaints and Appeals. The regulations establish meaningful processes for resolution of complaints and appeals. Similar processes already exist for resolution of disputes arising in fee-for-service settings.

Internal Appeals. The regulations provide for the establishment of internal (plan-level) appeal processes, with explicit timeframes for both prior authorizations and resolution of appeals at the plan level. Both the Medicare and Medicaid regulations establish a process for expedited review of prior authorizations and resolution of appeals by plans in emergency or urgent care situations. Extensions for both the standard and expedited timeframes are possible only under limited circumstances.

External Appeals. The Bill of Rights provides that an appeal process include an independent system of external review, in order to ensure its fairness and accuracy. Medicare has long had this protection which includes a provision for expedited decisions in time-sensitive areas. Individuals who are dissatisfied with the determination of the independent external review entity have the right to pursue their claim for Medicare benefits further through an administrative review, including review by the Departmental Appeals Board and, ultimately, federal court.

The appeals process for Medicaid differs from the Bill of Rights in two significant ways. The Bill of Rights calls for the establishment of a sequential process of internal (plan-level) and external review. However, states are permitted to design their appeals systems so that individuals can appeal either sequentially or simultaneously to the state's fair hearing process, which otherwise serves as the independent external review entity. Second, the state fair hearing process, which serves a docket of programs and issues much broader than Medicaid managed care, currently has timeframes that are not consistent with the timeframes for internal review by Medicaid managed care plans; in addition, there is no provision for expedited review.

Federal bill of Rights Web site-*http://www.hhs.gov/news/press/1999pres/990412.html*

The Hospital During Off-Hours

`David J. Shulkin, M.D.

What Can I Do to Make My Care Safer When I am in the Hospital on Nights and Weekends?

Most patients are admitted to hospitals at night or on weekends. In fact, between 60 and 70% of all admissions occur during these off-hours. Numerous studies have shown that outcomes of care may not be as good when people are admitted during nights and weekends. Most people think of hospitals as bustling places filled with doctors and nurses rushing around. The reality is that on these off-hours, hospitals can be sparsely staffed and many services that are available during normal workdays are not readily available.

Despite this stark reality, by following a few simple rules, patients and families can improve the off-hours experience in the hospital. In fact, following these seven rules may help safeguard your experience in the hospital.

Rule 1: Ask Questions Now

Talk with your doctor about a night and weekend plan in the event you need to be hospitalized. Ask and review these questions: Which hospital should you go to? How can you reach your doctor, or the backup doctor, while you are hospitalized? How can other hospital staff get access to your past medical information?

Rule 2: Investigate Physician Involvement

Find out which hospitals in your area have attending physicians on-site 24 hours a day. Ask whether these attending physicians include those in sub-specialties like anesthesia, emergency medicine, obstetrics, pediatrics and neonatology, and intensive care medicine.

Rule 3: Prepare Your Medical Information

Keep handy a list of your medical conditions, medications and doses, allergies, and important test results. If your physician's office keeps your medical record in digital format, ask the staff for a copy of it on a CD or DVD.

Rule 4: Don't Be Passive

If you have questions about your medical care, don't wait. Ask to speak to someone immediately. If you're not satisfied with the answers you receive, ask to speak to that person's supervisor.

Rule 5: Know Your Attending Physician

If you feel something is wrong in your care, always insist on speaking to the attending physician assigned to you. Staff physicians and physicians-in-training (also known as residents) provide excellent care at night, but you are entitled to speak with the attending physician, who is the senior doctor in charge of your care.

Rule 6: Escalate Issues

Remember the old adage, "The squeaky wheel gets the grease." If you have spoken with a supervisor and your concerns still haven't been resolved, ask to speak to someone at the next level. All hospitals have chain-of-command procedures through which problems are resolved. Unresolved issues escalate to a higher level in the organization. If an issue is serious, or potentially serious, you should not have to wait until the morning to get the proper attention.

Rule 7: Participate in the handoff

When caregivers change shifts, insist that the handoff of information take place at your bedside or in the presence of your proxy. For example, if you had a chest x-ray in the evening but the film had not yet been officially read or reviewed, a doctor on a later shift may be the one who is responsible for following up on that reading and checking to be sure that the result is okay. A "handoff" is when the doctor from the first shift instructs the doctor on the next shift to be sure to check the result of the x-ray. Many errors occur when healthcare professionals leave the hospital and fail to transmit important information to the caregivers who take their place. Being present or asking the doctors on each shift about the handoff can reinforce that these communications were completed.

Unless you work in hospitals, it can be difficult to understand how these complex organizations work. Yet knowing something about the differences between days and nights can turn out to be very useful in navigating one's way through the recovery process.

Some Final Thoughts on Off-Hours Care

Often coming to the hospital on nights or weekends is not something that can be prevented. If properly prepared, there is no reason to be overly concerned about the hospital on off-hours. However, there is even more of an imperative for patients and families to be active participants in their care during these times. The single most important issue during off-hours is to have a good understanding of which attending physician is accountable for you and to establish a treatment plan with your physician. If complications do occur, or your situation changes at any time of day in the hospital you should make sure that your attending physician is aware of the events.

Reference:

Shulkin D. Like Night and Day—Shedding Light on Off-Hours Care. New England Journal of Medicine 2008:358(20):2092-2094.

Going Home

Preparing for Your Discharge

Fran Silverman, LCSW, ACSW and
Alicia Tennenbaum, LCSW, ACSW

How can I prepare for my discharge?

Being in the hospital, whether planned or unexpected can be stressful and upsetting. Although some come to the hospital for a planned procedure, many hospitalizations are unplanned. In 2005, 43% of patients nationwide, were admitted to the hospital from the Emergency Department according to statistics from the Department of Health and Human Services. Therefore, it is important to have an understanding of what to expect, what information you will need to know, both while in the hospital and upon your return to the community. This chapter will prepare you in the event of both: an unexpected hospitalization and a planned procedure.

You must keep in mind that an important principle for hospital staff is that plans for your discharge begin on the day of your admission. As soon as your doctor determines that you no longer need treatment in the hospital, you will be discharged. Staying in the hospital longer than is necessary can lead to a variety of infections, loss of physical strength and can affect your mental health.

How can I participate in my own care?

It is important for you and your family to be active participants in your care and in your discharge. Although the expectation is that you will be making decisions about your own care, it is essential to plan ahead in case you are unable to make your own decisions. The best time to discuss your wishes about your health care is when you are healthy, comfortable and able to think clearly. Who do you trust to speak for you in the event you are unable to speak for yourself? That person should be appointed your Health Care Proxy. (See copy of Health Care Proxy in the Appendix). Designating a proxy assumes that you have discussed your wishes regarding things like artificial life support, tube feedings and even the kind of care you should receive upon discharge. Some people draw up a living will. This is something you can discuss with your attorney, but a health care proxy is acceptable anywhere. Once completed, you should give your health care proxy a copy, as well as your primary care doctor. Keep your copy with your other important papers and a copy with you in your wallet. Health Care Proxy forms are available in many office supply stores, online and at your hospital or doctor's office. You can even write it on your own stationery, with your signature and a witness' signature, but completing the actual form would be best.

But, let's assume now that you can speak for yourself. What do you need to know in order to participate in your care and discharge?

Who will talk to me about my discharge?

In most hospitals, there are designated staff that focus primarily on discharge planning. Social work has long been the leader in this, but in some hospitals, you may have a case manager, a discharge planner or other health care provider who assumes this role. Of course the doctors, nurses and other health care providers will be talking to you about your discharge, but the social worker will ultimately make the final plan with you and your family.

What are the common questions I will be asked?

Upon meeting you, the social worker will complete an assessment, gathering key information about you and your family. Some of the questions may not seem relevant to the reason you are in the hospital, but they are all important in developing a safe and realistic plan with you. Some of the questions are:

- Who do you live with?
- Who should we be talking to about your discharge?
- How do you financially support yourself?
- What insurance do you have?
- Do you use special equipment such as a wheelchair or walker?
- Are there entry stairs or stairs within your home?
- Do you have a psychiatric and/or substance abuse history?
- Have you been physically, sexually or emotionally hurt by someone close to you?
- Will you need help at home?
- Can you go home directly from the hospital?

Asking for help

Many people believe that when they leave the hospital they will need help, because they had a procedure or are in pain, and feel they cannot perform their usual activities. When asking for help, you must be specific about the kind of help you are asking for. Asking for help with housekeeping is a different kind of request than asking for help with personal care, such as bathing and toileting. These kinds of services are called home care.

One cannot talk about home care without also discussing insurance. Regardless of what you "want" or "need," your insurance will determine the kind of care that will be covered upon discharge. Most managed care companies follow the Medicare guidelines, so we will refer to the Medicare requirements when discussing home care. In the next section, we provide explanations and examples of the different types of home care you may be eligible to receive.

What types of home care are there?

Patients often wonder, "Who is going to help me when I get home?" In order to qualify for home care under Medicare, you must have a "skilled need." A skilled need is one that requires the services of a nurse, physical therapist, occupational therapist, or speech therapist. Think of it in terms of a skill that a family member or neighbor cannot perform. Some examples of a skilled need for a nurse at home are wound care; needing intravenous therapy, short term monitoring of your blood pressure; heart rate, and temperature, and diabetic teaching. Your social worker can discuss home care agencies covered under your specific insurance, so that you choose the agency you prefer. Once you have chosen an agency, the social worker will make a referral to that agency. Generally, the day after discharge, a nurse from the agency will come to your home to evaluate you and develop a "care plan." Under some managed care companies, it may take two or more days for the nurse to come for the initial evaluation.

Tasks such as bathing and getting dressed are done by a home health aide. In addition to these personal care needs, tasks such as meal preparation and light cleaning may also be done by the home health aide. Some tasks that a home health aide cannot perform are giving medications, taking care of other family members, heavy duty cleaning, tube feedings and intravenous antibiotics. Be aware that many insurance companies, with the exception of Medicare, will not cover home health aides. If it is determined that you require a home health aide in addition to a nurse or therapist, Medicare may provide a home health aide up to five days a week, Monday through Friday, four hours each day. Keep in mind that Medicare home care is time limited and will not last for a very long time.

The agency nurse is the main contact person who will advise you on how long you will have the services and for how many times per week. The nurse also supervises the home health aide and ensures that the care plan is followed.

Medicare requires that you are homebound in order to receive home care. For example, if you are able to get to the grocery store, or the hair salon, you are not considered homebound and therefore are ineligible for services. Additionally, if you go to outpatient physical therapy, Medicare will not consider you homebound and will not provide nursing or aide service.

Even though your doctor may promise you help at home, you may not be entitled to the kind of help you are asking for under your insurance or under the criteria set by the home care agency. A few examples of agency criteria are a safe home environment, how well you are able to follow the treatment recommendations, and if you have other people to assist in your care.

If your insurance does not cover a home health aide, or you will need to hire a home health aide beyond what Medicare provides, the social worker can provide you with a list of agencies that you can contact and privately hire to assist you. If you require medical equipment such as a wheelchair or walker, this can be ordered by the social worker or physical therapist while you are still in the hospital. Medicare will pay 80% of the approved amount (Medicare Rights Center, Volume 7, Issue 18, May 5, 2008)

What if I need treatment in another facility before going home?

If you are not strong enough to go home or you have had a major change in your medical/physical condition, you may be advised that you need rehabilitation (rehab). There are two choices. One is called acute rehab and the other is sub-acute rehab. Acute rehab is in a hospital setting and provides three hours a day of intensive physical therapy. Sub-acute rehab is in a skilled nursing facility, sometimes called a nursing home, and provides less intensive therapy: one to two hours a day. Just as with home care, insurance will dictate which in-network facility they will approve, what level of care and for how long you can stay. Each of these rehab facilities have criteria for admission, related to how well and how far you can walk, and how much therapy will help you return to the community. Your diagnosis will also be a factor for eligibility to an acute rehab center.

In planning a discharge to a facility, you will be asked to select at least five choices. Your social worker can discuss the variety of facilities that are appropriate for you. If you need to stay for a long period of time at a sub-acute facility, they will ask you about your finances to determine if you are eligible for Medicaid, which covers long-term care, called *custodial care*. The social worker completes the forms that the facilities require. Remember that friends and members of family can and should visit the facilities before you go, to make sure they are acceptable to you.

You may not have a lot of time to visit the facilities because patients must be discharged as soon as they are medically stable. This means that patients may not be able to wait for their first choice and may be discharged to the facility with the first available bed. You can have the application sent to as many places as you want, but when a bed is offered the hospital can discharge you.

What are your rights as a patient?

You are entitled to be informed of the date of your discharge, at a minimum of 24 hours before you are scheduled to go. If you think you are being discharged too soon, or that your discharge plan is unsafe, you can appeal your discharge, remaining in the hospital until a decision is reached. Hospital staff can guide you on how to appeal your discharge. After you notify the independent review organization that handles appeals, the hospital forwards your medical records to them. This decision is usually made within 24 hours and the review organization will notify you of the decision. If your appeal is denied and the hospital's decision to discharge is upheld, you will be liable for the hospital bill, beginning noon the day after you are notified of the denial. Medicare patients will receive a specific, written notice that discusses discharge appeal, entitled "An Important Message from Medicare About Your Rights."

Upon discharge, you should receive a copy of your discharge summary/instructions, which can be written by several of your providers: the social worker, the nurse and the doctor. The social worker's discharge summary will include the names and telephone numbers of all referrals made for you. The summaries written by doctors and nurses will include instructions for you to follow when you get home, a list of the medications you will be taking, and any follow up medical appointments that you require. It is important to keep these papers in a safe and readily accessible place once you are back in the community in case you need to refer to them.

Getting Home from the Hospital

It is a good idea to have a friend or family member present when you are being discharged. They can act as a "second set of eyes and ears" when you are given your discharge instructions, to ensure that once home everything is recalled correctly. It also makes sense to have a family member or friend take you home from the hospital. Let someone close to you help as you may feel weak, nervous about leaving, overwhelmed with the instructions you just received and taking care of yourself. If you cannot get home in a car or taxi cab, there are ambulettes which are "medical mini-vans," and are wheelchair accessible. This form of transportation is not covered by most insurance plans, but they are relatively inexpensive and can be ordered by the social worker in advance.

Have cash on hand to pay for the trip home. The ambulette driver will assist you into your home. Ambulances are used when there is a medical necessity, such as oxygen use, or your condition dictates that you cannot sit up but must lie down on a stretcher. If your insurance deems an ambulance is necessary it will be covered. If they do not, ambulances are quite costly to pay on your own. Your community may also have special programs that transport elderly and disabled individuals to and from the hospital and medical appointments. Once again, your social worker would be able to discuss this with you.

If you choose to be transferred to another hospital, that transport will not be covered by your insurance. Your insurance will only cover transfer to another hospital, if the company requests it because the hospital you are in is not in their network, or some treatment or procedure you need is only available at another hospital.

Letting The Hospital Know About My Experience

Hospitals, such Beth Israel Medical Center, strive to provide the very best care for each and every patient. In order to accomplish this, it is important that patients and families let us know about their hospital experience. There is a variety of forums to do this. In the hospital itself, there may be a Patient Representative Department, or Ombudsman's Office, where staff assist in addressing any difficulties you might be experiencing and ensuring that your rights are upheld.

Once discharged, many hospitals have surveys mailed to you where you can give both praise and constructive criticism. These results are now available online (see Resources for listings of these survey results). Whether or not the results are online, the hospital needs to hear from you about what needs to be improved. And for the things that went well, it is important that we know that, too, as we can acknowledge the staff that contributed to your positive experience and continue to provide excellent quality of care.

A more direct and personal approach to giving feedback is writing letters—you can write to the people who helped you, or you can write to the CEO or President of the hospital to let them know about your experience.

HELPFUL TIPS

- Discuss your living will, advanced directives with your family, health care proxy and primary care doctor so that everyone knows your wishes
- Keep an updated folder containing information that will be important to know when you are hospitalized:

  o your emergency contact information
  o copies of insurance cards
  o updated list of medications you are taking

o   list of preferred medications under your prescription plan
o   allergies
o   your doctors' names and telephone numbers
o   health care proxy, living will, power of attorney
o   name and phone number of your home care agency if you are receiving services

- Know about your specific insurance coverage.

o   Does it cover home care services?
o   Do you need to contact your insurance carrier when you are hospitalized?
o   What health related facilities are in your network?

- Investigate your local resources, such as your place of worship, senior centers and community centers to determine if they provide any assistance in the community after a hospitalization.
- Ask your friends and relatives who may have used home care services about which agencies they have used and whether they would recommend them
- Visit skilled nursing facilities

o   Going on the weekends, when there are fewer supervisory staff around, helps you see how the staff take care of the patients "on their own"
o   Also, going on the weekend gives you the opportunity to talk to other family members who visit on the weekends to get their perspectives
o   Look around—how does the place look? Are the patients clean, dressed, active? Does the facility have a bad odor?
o   How does the staff relate to the patients? Do they know the patients' names?
o   Ask to see the specific floor you or your relative may be on
o   Can your primary doctor have privileges there? If not, are there doctors on site?
o   What other medical specialists are available: i.e. psychiatry, podiatry, dental? How often are they available?
o   What special services do they offer on site if, for example, you had a wound that needed specialized care? Or if you needed to be on ventilator to help you breathe or needed dialysis?
o   Can you choose which hospital you want to go to if you become ill while at the facility?

    o   How would you get to specialist appointments?
    o   What religious services are available?
    o   Is there physical therapy on the weekends?
    o   Are there specific visiting hours?

- Look into long term care and catastrophic insurance. Sometimes it is worthwhile.
- You may want to research your eligibility for Medicaid, a government assistance program, based on your income and resources, which pays for a range of medical services. Keep in mind that Medicaid benefits differ from state to state.
- Consult an elder law attorney if you have concerns about your assets and your long term care planning, including Medicaid eligibility.

RESOURCES

- For questions about health insurance choices, Medicare rights and protections, payment denials or appeals, complaints about care or treatment, Medicare bills:

  Medicare Rights Center's Consumer Hotline 800-333-4114, available between 9 a.m. and 6 p.m., Eastern Time, Monday through Friday— **Medicare Rights Center**—520 Eighth Avenue, North Wing, 3rd Floor, New York, NY 10018, Phone: 212-869-3850, Fax: 212-869-3532 or 110 Maryland Ave, NE, Suite 112, Washington, DC 20002, Phone: 202-544-5561, Fax: 202-544-5549

- For information related to all Medicare benefits, comparisons between hospitals as well as comparisons between nursing homes and on-line individual hospital survey results: *www.medicare.gov*
- For information related to benefits under Medicare and Medicaid, as well as information on health care facilities: *www.cms.hhs.gov*
- For information about Medicaid eligibility in your state, visit the local Department of Social Services
- For comparisons between hospitals: *www.hospitalcompare.hhs.gov*
- To locate and select home care agencies—National Association for Home Care and Hospice (NAHC) *www.nahc.org.*
- For information on hospitals and nursing homes in your area, contact your local Department of Health
- For information on community services for the aging population in your area, contact your local Department for the Aging

Rehabilitation after Hospitalization

Kevin Weiner, M.D. and Christine Hinke, M.D.

Advances in healthcare have resulted in many positive changes for patients that suffer from accidents, sudden illnesses or complications of chronic diseases. Patients recovering in hospitals may develop a loss of functional abilities, including the ability to walk, talk, or perform basic tasks, such as eating, dressing, and bathing. A rehabilitation program is often necessary to regain these functions.

A basic knowledge of the field of rehabilitation medicine and the types of services available is an important part of choosing the most appropriate post-illness treatment plan.

What is a Physiatrist?

A Physiatrist, or Rehabilitation Physician, is a physician specializing in Physical Medicine and Rehabilitation, who is trained to evaluate the disability that can occur as the result of trauma, illness, its complications and sometimes, its treatments. The physiatrist's job is to evaluate the function of the patient while keeping medical issues in mind and develop a comprehensive treatment plan to return the patient to the highest level of function possible.

Physiatrists are physicians, either MDs or DOs, and not physical therapists or doctors of physical therapy. You should always inquire about the credentials of the rehabilitation team members involved in your care.

What Rehabilitation Options are Available after an Illness or Injury?

There are several different types of rehabilitation settings that can be considered after being hospitalized. The type of rehabilitation that is most appropriate depends on a variety of factors, including pre-illness function, expectations for recovery, motivation, and even insurance coverage.

Acute inpatient rehabilitation facilities are specialized units, or sometimes separate hospitals, which offer comprehensive treatment programs for patients with disabilities. Care in this type of facility must be directed by a specialist in Physical Medicine and Rehabilitation. The patients must receive a minimum of 3 hours of therapy, including at least 2 different types of therapy. The nursing staff should be specially trained to assist patients to achieve their goals. These facilities offer short-term rehabilitation, which can vary from 5 to 35 days depending on diagnosis and disability. Most patients are discharged home from these facilities.

Subacute inpatient rehabilitation facilities are specialized units in nursing homes, which offer rehabilitation at a lower level than acute inpatient rehabilitation facilities. The rehabilitation is directed by a physician; however, the physician is not required to have any training in rehabilitation medicine. Basic nursing care is provided as needed; however, rehabilitation nursing is not required. Patients are given a minimum of 1 hour of therapy daily, and may only consist of one type of therapy. These facilities offer long-term rehabilitation, which can vary from weeks to months. A lower percentage of patients are discharged home from these facilities.

Home rehabilitation services can be provided by a visiting nurse service. The amount and type of services available is often dependent on insurance coverage. This option is available to patients who are functioning well enough to be discharged from the hospital back to an appropriate home setting, but who are not capable of being transported to and from an outpatient therapy area.

Outpatient rehabilitation services can be provided in hospital outpatient areas or in community locations. The amount and type of services is determined by prescriptions written by the treating physicians, and insurance coverage. This option is available to patients who are well enough to be discharged home and well enough to tolerate transportation to and from the therapy area.

Are Rehabilitation Services covered by all Insurance Policies?

No.

Rehabilitation services are always considered elective, meaning that the services are not necessary to preserve the life of a patient. Coverage for rehabilitation services is based upon your policy's specific benefits and it is important for you to know what your benefits are. Changes in your policy, whether made by you or your employer, can affect which rehabilitation benefits can or will be covered.

All Medicare and Medicaid policies, including managed plans, have rehabilitation benefits. Managed plans require authorizations for rehabilitation services. Commercial plans, whether managed or not, are not required to have rehabilitation benefits. If you have rehabilitation benefits, the benefits may be limited to certain types of services and may require authorization.

How do I know what my Insurance Covers?

Many people are not familiar with the specific benefits of their insurance policies until they need healthcare services. It is a good idea to familiarize yourself with your benefits and review them yearly. However, if you are in the hospital and are not sure about your benefits, speak to your social worker. The social worker can assist you by having your insurance company contacted and checking your "benefits and eligibility."

If I think I need therapy, what should I do?

Ask your doctor.

Therapy services require a physician's prescription. If your doctor is not available, speak with the nurse or social worker, so that he/she can contact your doctor about your request.

I have been told that I am ready to be discharged to an inpatient Rehabilitation facility. How can I tell if I am choosing a facility with good quality?

First, ask your doctor. Your doctor may have experience with local rehabilitation facilities and may prefer one facility over another. Your physician may be able to continue seeing you during your rehabilitation stay at certain facilities, but not others. This may be a consideration in choosing a facility.

Also, you need to know what type of rehabilitation you will be receiving. Different levels of rehabilitation will offer different services. If the facility is not located in the hospital, it may be helpful to have a family member visit the facility before you choose it.

You should ask about the types of services available, the training of the doctors and therapy staff, and percentage of patients discharged home after rehabilitation. If you have special needs, such as food preferences/restrictions; language or sign-language needs, access to specific medical treatments, like dialysis or radiation treatment, your choice of facilities may be limited.

What can I expect during my acute inpatient Rehabilitation hospitalization?

If you are admitted to an acute inpatient rehabilitation facility, you will be evaluated by a Rehabilitation specialist (a Physiatrist), who will evaluate your medical and functional needs and set up a treatment program, designed specifically for you, that consists of any appropriate medical treatments, rehabilitation nursing, and therapy services.

You will receive a minimum of three hours of therapy, which must be combination of at least two of the following: Physical Therapy; Occupational Therapy; and/or Speech Language Pathology. The amount and type of therapy will depend on the prescriptions written by the Physiatrist.

Your therapy team will consist of a Physiatrist, Rehabilitation Nurses, a Physical Therapist, an Occupational Therapist, and a Social Worker. Depending on your needs, your team may also include a Speech Language Pathologist for any speech or swallowing problems; an Orthotist-Prosthetist for any brace or artificial limb needs; and/or a Psychologist for any psychological needs.

On admission, you become an important member of your own rehabilitation team, and will be expected to assist in your own recovery process. You will be expected to participate in as much of your own care as possible, even if it is difficult for you. You will be expected to participate in all required activities. In fact, failure to participate may require you to be discharged, even if you have not reached your goals.

The members of your team will evaluate your ability to perform 18 specific functions, called "FIM items." Your abilities will be evaluated on admission, throughout your stay, and upon discharge. Your performance of these functions will help to guide your therapy and determine your needs upon discharge.

How can I get the most from my Acute Inpatient Rehabilitation Admission?

Set Goals: Your rehabilitation team will set goals for you and should explain them to you. The team should also ask you what your goals are and should try to incorporate any additional goals into your treatment plan. If your goals are unrealistic, the team should discuss the reasons why, and help you focus on realistic ones.

Participate: You have chosen to be admitted for inpatient rehabilitation and full participation will ensure an optimal outcome. No one else can do your therapy for you. Some activities or tasks may seem silly, difficult, or unimportant to you. You may be tired, frustrated, or depressed. However, trust that your team is guiding you through the rehabilitation process and will not ask you to perform tasks to embarrass you, hurt you, or waste your time. Everything you are asked to do has a purpose. Don't be afraid to ask what it is. Make sure you have comfortable clothing and supportive shoes available to use during therapy. Hospital gowns and slippers are not adequate for full participation.

Communicate with your team and ask questions: Your team cannot help you if you don't let them know about your needs or concerns. You must report any pain or new symptoms immediately. Rehabilitation is really a learning process and asking questions will help you get the most out of the experience. Write down your questions if you think of them and the person you want to ask is not available at that time. Ask for written answers or information if you don't think you will remember the answers. Remember, there is no such thing as a stupid question!

Do your "homework": Your team should give you exercises or activities to do on your own, with the assistance of the nursing staff, or even with the assistance of family members and visitors. Techniques learned in therapy require practice and remember, "Practice makes perfect." Rehabilitation nurses are trained to assist you to use techniques learned in therapy. You are expected to practice those techniques when you are not in therapy, in order for you to eventually be able to do them with the least amount of help at home.

Know your discharge plan: Your doctor should discuss your discharge plan with you on admission. You should be told approximately how long your stay is expected to be, what goals you are expected to achieve, and what services you are likely to need upon discharge. Your team will meet at least once a week to discuss your progress, and should update you on any changes to your treatment plan, goals, or discharge date or destination. You should be encouraged to go to your own team conference.

I am afraid I might fall. How can I prevent falls?

Prevention of falls by patients in a hospital is a priority for everyone on staff at every hospital. All hospitals must evaluate you for "fall risk" and develop a fall prevention treatment plan. However, you can assist the staff in preventing falls by remembering a few simple suggestions:

1. Use your call bell to ask for assistance to get in and out of bed; walk around the room; use the bathroom, etc.
2. Remind staff members about your limitations, even if you think he/she "knows" them.
3. Do not ask family members or visitors to assist you, unless they have been trained by the staff to do so.
4. Do not physically assist other patients and risk injury to yourself. If necessary, use your call bell to ring for assistance for another patient in need.

Can my doctor still take care of me when I am admitted to the Acute Rehabilitation Service?

If your rehabilitation facility is located within the same hospital, then, yes. However, your doctor would be a consultant during your rehabilitation stay, and work with your Physiatrist to take care of you. Other consultants from your acute hospital stay may also continue to monitor you on the rehabilitation unit.

If you are admitted to a different facility, your doctor(s) may not be able to remain on your case. You should ask to be sure.

What happens if I develop a complication from a medical illness and I am on the acute inpatient rehabilitation unit?

Part of the reason that patients are admitted to inpatient rehabilitation facilities is that those patients are at risk for certain types of complications. Physiatrists are trained to anticipate and try to prevent some common complications of patients who are newly disabled. In addition, they are trained to recognize other complications quickly to start treatment as soon as possible.

Certain complications are known to occur and treatment should be considered to prevent them. These include such things as bladder infections, blood clots in the leg veins, and bedsores. A prevention plan should be a part of the treatment prescribed by the Physiatrist and a care-plan is developed by the rehabilitation nurses. You should be educated by the nursing staff about your specific plan. Ask about your plan if you are not told about it. If you do develop these complications, they can be treated during the rehabilitation stay and rarely affect your ability to participate in therapy.

Patients can also develop new conditions or changes in their condition that require care from other specialists. Consultants will be called by the Physiatrist whenever necessary and will assist in your medical care as you continue your rehabilitation.

Other, more serious complications, can also occur and may require higher level care or not allow safe participation in the rehabilitation program. These types of complications include such conditions as heart attacks, strokes, blood clots in the lungs, pneumonia, severe infections, and abnormal heart rhythms. You would require transfer back to the acute hospital for these types of conditions

Rehabilitation Medicine Resources for Patients

American Academy of PM&R: *http://www.aapmr.org/condtreat/what.htm*
National Institutes of Health: *http://www.cc.nih.gov/rmd/*

Sharing Stories
On Being a Patient

Telling a story can be powerful. In fact, people in need of medical care are eager to hear about others' experiences and lessons. In times of need we are all desirous for information. Learning how a friend or relative was helped by a doctor or treatment can be useful and comforting. Similarly, we've all heard stories of patients who have suffered as a result of error. These anecdotes are powerful and can be important lessons for us all. Medical error does not discriminate between the rich and poor or young and old. It is something that requires all of us to be aware of and guard against. It's for this reason that telling our stories is important.

Fortunately, the vast majority of patients never experience an error and do not have problems in the hospital. However, preventable error is still all too common. Hearing about other patients problems has a purpose. It's not meant to scare people, but rather to make the point that patients and their families must be aware and active participants in their healthcare recovery. The objective of involving patients in the care process is not to have them become as knowledgeable about the disease process as the doctor, but rather to be involved in those parts of the system that may be high risk.

As we continue our quest to make healthcare safer, I hope to enlist you in the efforts by asking you to share your own stories and experiences. By doing so, you'll be part of the solutions that will be designed and implemented in upcoming years. I'd also be eager to hear from you with any additional questions (my email address is listed below) that you may have had during a healthcare interaction. As the old adage goes "there are no such thing as stupid questions". I anticipate that by sharing your stories and questions that there will likely be a second edition of "Questions Patients Need to Ask" in the offing. As long as there are new ideas to making healthcare safer, I hope that together we can be part of this journey.

David J. Shulkin, M.D.
www.QuestionsPatientsAsk.com

About the Editor
David J. Shulkin, MD

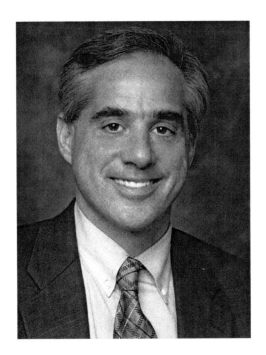

David J. Shulkin, M.D. was recently named as one of the "One Hundred Most Powerful People in Healthcare" by Modern Healthcare. Dr. Shulkin is President and Chief Executive Officer of Beth Israel Medical Center in New York City. He previously served in numerous physician leadership roles including the Chief Medical Officer of the University of Pennsylvania Health System, Temple University Hospital, the Medical College of Pennsylvania Hospital, and the Hospital of the University of Pennsylvania. Dr. Shulkin has served in academic positions including the Chairman of Medicine and Vice Dean at Drexel University School of Medicine. As an entrepreneur Dr. Shulkin founded and served as the Chairman and CEO of DoctorQuality, Inc one of the first consumer orientated sources of information for quality and safety in healthcare. Dr. Shulkin has been on the editorial boards of numerous journals including the Journal of the American Medical Association. Currently the editor of Hospital Physician, he also serves on the editorial boards of the Journal of Patient Safety, the Journal of Clinical Outcomes Management and the Journal of Disease Management.

Dr. Shulkin is a board-certified internist, a fellow of the American College of Physicians, Professor of Medicine at Albert Einstein College of Medicine and a Senior Fellow at the Leonard Davis Institute in Health Economics at the University of Pennsylvania. He received his medical degree from the Medical College of Pennsylvania, his internship at Yale University School of Medicine, and a residency and Fellowship in General Medicine at the University of Pittsburgh Presbyterian Medical Center. He had advanced training in outcomes research and economics as a Robert Wood Johnson Foundation Clinical Scholar at the University of Pennsylvania. Dr. Shulkin has received numerous awards and was named one of the country's top Health care leaders for the next century by Modern Healthcare, the International Leader in Health Care Award by the Healthcare Forum and in 2008 was selected as the 12th most powerful physician executive in America by Modern Physician.

Shulkin, David J., M.D.
610.696   Questions Patients Need to Ask
S   Getting the Best Healthcare.
           Meherrin Regional Library

DEC 1 4 2009

Meherrin Regional Library System
133 W. Hicks St.
Lawrenceville, VA 23868

Breinigsville, PA USA
17 September 2009
224271BV00002B/76/P

9 781436 367592